THE ANTISOCIAL CHILD
His Family
and
His Community

THE LANGLEY PORTER

CHILD PSYCHIATRY SERIES

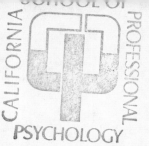

THE ANTISOCIAL CHILD
His Family
and
His Community

Edited by
S. A. Szurek, M.D., and I. N. Berlin, M.D.

The Langley Porter Child Psychiatry Series
Clinical Approaches to Problems of Childhood
Volume 4

SCIENCE AND BEHAVIOR BOOKS, INC.
577 College Avenue, Palo Alto, California 94306

THE ANTISOCIAL CHILD
His Family and His Community
Second printing, February 1970
Copyright © 1969 by Science and Behavior Books, Inc.
Printed in the United States of America. All rights reserved. This book, or parts thereof, may not be reproduced in any form without permission of the publisher.

Library of Congress Card Catalog Number: 68-54535

ISBN: 0-8314-0020-X

PREFACE

This volume, the three that preceded it, and the one that will follow result from the encouragement we have received from our own students and graduates to make available to them our papers, published and unpublished, past and present. There has also been a continuing demand for reprints no longer available, of papers published in journals no longer in existence. In addition, it is our hope that the materials we have found useful and appreciated in our own teaching may find sympathetic reading by, and be of use to, other professional persons concerned with children and their clinical problems.

An effort has been made throughout to express ideas in language that is understandable to many professions. Occasionally, in the interests of precision, a concept has been discussed in psychoanalytic terms; however, we find that many of these expressions have already passed into the popular language. (Should the reader wish further explanation of any of the terms he encounters, he will find English and English, A Comprehensive Dictionary of Psychological and Psychoanalytic Terms, or Hinsie and Campbell, Psychiatric Dictionary, helpful.)

It will be clear to the reader that each paper must be judged in terms of the period during which it was written. Yet, in human affairs and dynamic processes—especially in personal, emotionally important events—history does not change much from one generation to the next. Sometimes social problems have a way of repeating themselves on a more massive scale, as the current increase in population is seen now to complicate further the problems for both parents and children. Wars and economic difficulties, with concomitant intensification of strain, also continue to occur. One of the points at issue is that conflicts of parents continue to affect personality development of their children over a span of many generations. Hence papers written over the past twenty to twenty-five years continue to be in large measure relevant for the present generation. This remains true for us—after reading some of the older papers—despite the developments the last quarter-century has wrought in social organization by technological developments, changes in international relations, and changes in relations between ethnic groups in our society. The depersonalization common today makes an understanding of parent-child relations even more important now than in the past.

All the papers are published in substantially their original form. However, to avoid repetition and increase readability, minor editing and abridgement have been done. Several papers that appeared in Volume 1, Learning and Its Disorders, have been included here as well, since many interested professionals in the fields of correction and law enforcement may not have access to the earlier volume.

We should like to take this opportunity to thank Mary Polf, Carol Hite, and Elaine Hines for their considerable help in preparation of the manuscript. We also wish to express our appreciation to friends and colleagues who have contributed to the Child Psychiatry Fund of the University of California San Francisco Medical Center, helping to make publication of this series possible.

FOREWORD

To the child psychiatrist and to his associated social scientists who deal clinically with the expressions of severe antisocial behaviors by their child patients, the literature in this field that might come to their aid has suffered from very definite shortcomings and hiatuses in applicability.

In the first place they have seen advanced in the past three decades only a very few theoretical notions as to the etiology of such behaviors—theories that are original and that in their application "psychotherapywise" seem to be productive of good clinical results.

Secondly, the few new theories advanced have neglected those factors in "dynamic explanation" that in a larger sense extend beyond the strictly intrapsychic problems of the child himself. Thus, they exclude those important factors that evolve from the problems that exist in the most significant purveyors of attitudes and values for the growing child—the parents.

Thirdly, to present-day clinical practitioners, few of the contributions to the scientific literature have attuned their theoretical constructs and practical applications to the world and work of the new comprehensive mental health centers for children and their parents—including specifically their experience in the incidence, treatment, and control of child antisocial behavior.

This volume seems to me to correct all of these shortcomings. Hitherto, the authors—Dr. Szurek, Dr. Berlin, and their associates—have been content to have their theoretical positions, observations, and lucid outlines of the varied roles of the various practitioners in the field published in articles scattered through several scientific journals. In the present work these papers are assembled in a unified treatise.

To my own personal delight—and I am sure to that of other workers in the field—the theoretical structure promulgated by Dr. Szurek and Adelaide Johnson was, and continues to be, not only highly valuable for individual application, but also heuristic in that it leads to newer discoveries, newer observations of import, and newer, wider meaningful applications.

vii

As in other areas of child behavior on which these authors have written in the first three volumes of this series, they have in this present volume tenaciously and fruitfully followed a theoretical construct to make a lasting contribution to the literature dealing with the multiple problems of the antisocial child.

George E. Gardner, Ph.D., M.D.
Professor of Psychiatry
Harvard Medical School

INTRODUCTION

Delinquent, antisocial behavior of children has long been a concern of child psychiatrists. The establishment of the first child guidance clinics and the formation of the American Orthopsychiatric Association were stimulated by concern with increasing juvenile delinquency after the first world war. Early investigations indicated the complex nature of delinquency and the need not only to study and treat the child, but also to study the influences of family and immediate environment on the onset and exacerbations of delinquent behavior.

Today antisocial behavior is of increasing concern to communities both urban and suburban, and to the nation as a whole. It has become clear that there is a combination of sociological and intrafamilial influences which combine to produce the delinquent child. It has also become increasingly evident that the final common pathway, the mediating force of sociological conditions early in the child's life, is his parents. Thus, in recent years investigation, treatment, and rehabilitative efforts have encompassed study and work with the individual delinquent, his parents, the courts, and other community agencies involved with both child and parents.

Community mental health and mental health consultation with child-serving agencies have become increasingly important aspects of the activities of child psychiatrists. The juvenile courts, schools, and health and welfare agencies often seek help from a trained child psychiatrist to be more effective in their work with children and their families. Frequently the children and families who are most troublesome and time-consuming for these agency workers are those where antisocial problems are most prominent.

This volume includes papers on the genesis of antisocial behavior, some efforts at treatment, mental health consultation with the juvenile courts and other child serving agencies, as well as some papers on theoretical considerations of the nature of controls as they are related to the work of juvenile courts and of the mental health consultative process.

CONTRIBUTORS

BAIROS, MARION J., A.M., Certified Psychologist, Counseling and Testing Center, Stanford University; and Consulting Psychologists Associated, Palo Alto, California. Formerly at Child Guidance Clinic of Children's Hospital, San Francisco.

BERLIN, I.N., M.D., Professor of Psychiatry and Head, Division of Child Psychiatry, University of Washington School of Medicine, Seattle. Formerly Associate Clinical Professor of Psychiatry, University of California School of Medicine; and Coordinator of Training, Children's Service, Langley Porter Neuropsychiatric Institute, San Francisco.

BRUNSTETTER, R.W., M.D., Assistant Clinical Professor of Psychiatry, University of California School of Medicine; and Supervising Child Psychiatrist, Langley Porter Neuropsychiatric Institute, San Francisco.

GIANASCOL, A.J., M.D., most recently, Professor of Child Psychiatry, University of Pennsylvania Medical School and University of Pennsylvania Postgraduate School of Education. Formerly, Assistant Clinical Professor of Psychiatry, University of California School of Medicine, San Francisco. Now in private practice in Monterey, California.

KAPLAN, MAURICE, M.D., Director, South Coast Child Guidance Clinic, Costa Mesa, California. Formerly Director (half-time), Child Guidance Clinic of Children's Hospital, San Francisco; and Assistant Clinical Professor in Psychiatry, University of California School of Medicine, San Francisco.

LANGDELL, JOHN I., M.D., Assistant Clinical Professor of Psychiatry, University of California School of Medicine; and Supervising Child Psychiatrist, Langley Porter Neuropsychiatric Institute, San Francisco.

NATHAN, EDWARD, M.S.W., Lecturer and Consultant in Charge of Psychiatric Field Work for the School of Social Welfare, University of California, Berkeley.

RYAN, JOHN, M.D., Director, Child Guidance Clinic, Children's Hospital, San Francisco; and Assistant Clinical Professor of Psychiatry, University of California School of Medicine, San Francisco.

SUSSELMAN, SAMUEL, M.D., Associate Clinical Professor of Psychiatry, University of California School of Medicine; and Supervising Child Psychiatrist, Langley Porter Neuropsychiatric Institute, San Francisco.

SZUREK, S.A., M.D., Professor of Psychiatry, University of California School of Medicine; and Director, Children's Service, Langley Porter Neuropsychiatric Institute, San Francisco.

CONTENTS

SECTION ONE

GENESIS OF ANTISOCIAL BEHAVIOR IN CHILDREN

INTRODUCTION

The delinquent, hostile, aggressive child seems to behave in his particular ways in response to certain child-rearing practices of his parents. The unconscious conflicts of his parents as individuals, which are synthesized in his intimate experience with them in infancy and childhood, are the special concern of the papers which follow. Many writers on delinquency have expressed their debt to Adelaide Johnson and S. A. Szurek for their pioneering ideas contained in these papers.

CHILDHOOD ORIGINS OF
PSYCHOPATHIC PERSONALITY TRENDS*

S. A. Szurek

George Preston, in his delightful treatise on <u>Psychiatry for the Curious</u>, says, "We must always study one particular individual in one particular place at one particular time acting as the result of one particular series of causative factors. You could not draw pictures of 'delinquent children' but you could draw a picture of a boy stealing a watermelon out of a field in the summertime. You might be able to generalize a little about boys who stole watermelons . . . . Even if you did this, you would know nothing about the particular boy who stole the particular watermelon from the particular field. Human behavior, good, bad, indifferent, normal, insane (whatever those terms mean), is never carried out by boys, or girls, or men, or mankind, but always by a Particular Boy, Girl, Man or Woman in a certain place at some definite time and for a reason that is peculiar to that one and only that one person. You may make the averages for a hundred or a thousand individuals, but one of the big dangers of psychiatry is to believe that you can treat any particular human being on the basis of averages" (9, p. 37).

The simplicity of this statement still does not destroy its accuracy and truth. Its bearing, to my mind, on the topic of my discussion is that the need to group and classify people into nosologic entities has led to the difficulties, vagueness, and uncertainty with which the concept of "psychopathic personality" is enshrouded.

The dynamic conceptions current in psychiatric thought, as against the static descriptive efforts of Kraepelin and his followers, lead to several very obvious conclusions which bear upon the conception of this syndrome. First, the more thoroughly acquaint-

*Reprinted with permission from <u>Psychiatry</u>, 5:1-6, 1942. (Copyright is held by the William Alanson White Psychiatric Foundation, Inc. This article is a newly edited version.)

ed one becomes with the total behavior of any human being, the less easy it is to place him into a category, and the more one is aware of the specific meaning of his attitudes. One realizes nevertheless that the differences between that person and another person are largely quantitative. Second, the concept of personality becomes quite sharply defined as a person's more or less persistent set of tendencies to behave in a given manner in relation to other persons. The personality is then clearly seen as a more or less integrated system of attitudes toward the self, having its origin in the experiences with other persons. We see that although these attitudes are more or less modifiable throughout life the degree of this modifiability decreases with age and other factors, such as the absence of cultural opportunities and inadequate inherent assets. Conversely, it is also true that the attitudes which are experienced earliest in life are the most firmly integrated into the self and hence least easily modified by interpersonal influences occurring later in life. I am tempted to subscribe to the description of George Henry Mead (5) as the most succinct expression of all of psychodynamics, namely, the self is the taking of the attitude of the "generalized other" towards oneself. The only addition necessary is that this attitude toward the self is also in turn expressed towards others.

THE CONCEPT OF "PSYCHOPATHIC PERSONALITY"

If there is any agreement among those who have written[1] (2,6,7, 8) about "psychopathic personalities," it is in this: they are deficient in moral sense. But this deficiency is of a peculiar sort. It is not that they are unable intellectually to grasp the difference between "right" and "wrong," "good" or "bad." It is not that they do not very often act as if moved by, and apparently feel, some transient guilt, regret, or anxiety about some transgression against others—usually after the deed. It is rather that despite repeated experiences in which they have caused suffering to others and have been punished by their victims or authorities, at the next opportunity to gain similar immediate gratification of whatever impulses happen to control them, they are unable to inhibit or to postpone action, or to acquire satisfactions in culturally acceptable ways. It is this apparent urgency of their impulsive needs and this in-

---

[1]The paper by Partridge (8) contains an excellent review of the literature. There is also an earlier study by Partridge (7). The attention of the reader is invited to an excellent review of the literature and comments by Dunn (2). Another discussion of classification and some further suggestions are made by Menninger (6).

ability to modify their behavior despite usually educative experiences which leads many to consider their characteristics as a peculiar defect in constitution or structure[2] (1). It is also my impression that such persons possess a defect, but a defect in personality organization. It seems to me to be a defect which may be almost or even completely unmodifiable at a given age, or with the therapeutic means at the disposal of those responsible for their care and management—or for both reasons. It appears to me that the defect is in that general category of personality structures known as the conscience, that part of the self attained by positive, secure identifications with parents and their surrogates. The defect of conscience in these persons is a relative one—relative to a particular culture and relative in degree about any given interpersonal attitude. From this standpoint the concept of psychopathic personality could be extended to every so-called normal person in any culture, for on close study every person can be said to be psychopathic in the sense defined here, in some measure about one or another interpersonal attitude.

The culturally acquired self, the conscience or the superego, has also been defined in too discrete or too unitary a sense, and hence is at times confusing beyond usefulness as a concept. The whole problem is gaining some clarity and redefinition in the most recent attempts at reformulation. I should like to call attention to such efforts as those of Harry Stack Sullivan in his Conceptions of Modern Psychiatry (10) and of Abram Kardiner in The Individual and His Society (4). In those psychiatric clinics for children where

---

[2]Another explanation offered for essentially unmodifiable repetitive behavior leading to frustration of other, more important needs of a person is the hypothesis of the need for self-punishment. Although this tendency—ultimately an expression of revengeful motives against others turned on the self—may be an important determinant in those persons with a strong or well-developed conscience, it seems doubtful that it is an important factor in the persons described here. The distinction between a predominantly self-punitive act, which frustrates others as well as oneself in some way, and one which expresses a guiltless direct gratification of an impulse obviously depends on the presence of evidence of an actual conflict—that is, an alternation of attitudes—suffering, guilt, and attempts at restitution, for example, before or during the act. The assumption of an unconscious sense of guilt as a drive in a pattern of behavior leading to a need for punishment requires not only a study of the personality but also a careful reconstruction of the role of the total interpersonal milieu in which the particular behavior occurred.

close clinical study is <u>not</u> concentrated or limited to the child in question but includes the total interpersonal context, especially the integration of the parent and child, there has been a real contribution to the redefinition of the self in terms of dynamic processes. By dynamic processes I do not mean <u>only</u> those <u>within</u> the personality, so well elucidated by psychoanalytic investigation, but also those which occur <u>between</u> persons in any transient or durable integration.

CLINICAL EXAMPLE

A sketchy review of a recent case may illustrate more clearly my thesis:

A six-year-old boy was brought to the clinic by parents who were baffled by his extremely distractible hyperactivity, his inability to learn at school, destructiveness, pugnacity, and defiance of authority. The mother complained she did not dare leave him alone for a moment because she could not be certain what mischief would next attract him. Without warning and without apparent provocation he struck or kicked his playmates. On one occasion he struck his young cousin over the head with a hammer and continued his play apparently without concern or guilt. Yet his mother felt certain he was not malicious and did not bear any ill will toward children whom he laughingly chased with a knife. When a teacher gently reproved him for saying "shut up" to her, he kicked her in the shins, much to the chagrin of the mother who witnessed the incident. At the table the child indulged in throwing silverware at the china or at his brother and sister, rarely missing his target. The father felt he had a more obedient response from the boy than the mother did because he spanked him more frequently, but both parents insisted he never cried or showed that the punishment hurt. Similarly, when his provocativeness led to a gang retaliation by five of his schoolmates, he got up from his drubbing apparently without concern. According to his mother, he had been "the best baby" until he had learned to walk. Because he had not learned to talk until two or three and because his attention was so scattered during testing by a psychologist at another clinic, the parents were told it was impossible to state how retarded he was in mental development. They had become almost resigned to his "subnormal" condition.

During the visit at the clinic, whenever not directly engaged, he ran about the corridors noisily, shouted, and for brief periods investigated rooms, furniture, and equipment of the playroom. The psychologist found him unable to sit still long enough for his intelligence to be evaluated adequately, although he left the impression of being at least average in this respect. After repeating several short sentences correctly, he became more interested in the light switches and refused to repeat a longer test sentence. Several minutes later he sang out as if to himself, "We are going to have a good time in the country"—the sentence given him—without an error. In response to an effort at firmness by the psychologist, the boy yelled out and threatened to stab him in the face with a pencil. Eventually, the child ended the test by shouting, "You drive me nuts!" General examinations and examination of the nervous system revealed no organic disease, but the extreme, distractible hyperactivity led the psychiatrists to consider chronic encephalitis despite the lack of any history of acute illness.

The suggestion of the clinic staff that the parents place the boy in a suitable institution was not accepted. A progressive school refused to enroll him. In the first grade of the public school the child met a tolerant, accepting teacher, who reported that he seemed at the end of the year to be gaining some self-control, some "conscience about his errors," and was becoming somewhat more observant of common courtesies. Nevertheless, he rarely sat still, continually interrupted others, talked loudly, and exaggerated stories to keep the attention of others. He showed no timidity, delighting in sudden loud bursts of laughter. Although he appeared uninterested when taught, he seemed to the teacher to be retentive.

Re-examination at the clinic at intervals of seven months and two years after the first study yielded essentially the same results. An electroencephalographic examination on the last occasion was essentially inconclusive. At that time, however, his second grade teacher found him so unmanageable it was necessary to send him out of the classroom daily and to exclude him from class trips, though without effect. The mother still took him to school and called for him every day. His incorrigibility gave rise to much tension between the parents and the suburban school authorities, who requested an unbiased observer from the clinic to come to the school unannounced. As they put it, the boy was a "law unto himself."

About two years after the initial study, weekly psychiatric interviews with the mother were begun. After a few weeks of this régime she found it possible to reach the decision to place the boy in an excellent reeducational institution. It became very evident in these and subsequent visits what extreme neurotic interdependence had existed between mother and child. Despite the fifteen or sixteen interviews held thus far, information is still not complete concerning all the factors in the genesis of this parent-child adjustment, and although the maternal attitudes toward the boy are far from being essentially modified, enough evidence has been gathered to sketch the rough outlines of the picture.

The mother, a former school teacher who states she had no difficulties in rearing her two older children (a young man of twenty-one and a daughter of fifteen), became pregnant with the patient at the age of forty-two, at which time she felt her husband became progressively less interested in her. He was more interested in his books and business than in the social life of the community, which she states she enjoyed a great deal. She came to feel excluded from his affection, but at the same time unable to complain or find other satisfactions. The husband continued to support the family well and gave no other cause for complaint. It is fairly clear that she obtained an enormous amount of satisfaction in the care of the baby, applying toilet disciplines late and anticipating his every whim. The child progressively became the almost exclusive object of her devotion and extreme concern as she turned away from husband, her other children, and social engagements outside the home. Repeatedly she insists the boy became a problem to her only after he began to walk. She could not bear to allow him out of her sight at first, for fear something might happen to him and later for fear he would get into mischief and provoke retaliation or criticism—as he invariably proceeded to do.

She spent weeks considering removing the boy from the home and spent sleepless nights both before and after placing him in an institution. She knew better, yet suffered unbearable anxiety that he would not be adequately protected from harm in the boarding school, or that the school would soon find him actually mentally "subnormal" or too queer and uneducable to keep him. "He would run out in the street and be killed by an automobile. . . . He would climb out of the window and fall. . . . It is so silly, yet I can't help it," were her repeated complaints. Nevertheless, she experienced an enormous relief from tension and actually appeared to her relatives, as well as to the psychiatrist, to be a new woman within two weeks after placing him in the school.

She visits the school weekly even though not permitted to see the boy and is immeasurably relieved by short conversations with his teacher. She continuously vacillates between a wish to take him home and the knowledge that a lengthy period of separation is essential for them both. She requires repeated praise and encouragement from the school and from the psychiatrist that her decision is the correct one. Before making the bimonthly visits with her husband to see the boy at the school, she suffers agonies that he will either refuse to stay any longer or that he will feel unwanted by her. These anxieties continue despite reports of his improvement and her own direct observation that he seems content to remain. She continues to deny she is hurt or angered by his apparent indifference to her and his obvious preference for his teachers, and fails to report to the psychiatrist her amazement at the boy's ready obedience to his teacher. All the old fears recur at each interview, while simultaneously she insistently reports that she feels better, sees that the boy is calmer, that he is not subnormal, and that she understands more clearly every week what was wrong with herself and the boy.

A recent example she brought to the psychiatrist for discussion illustrates the extremely sado-masochistic relation between them. During a ride on a visit at the school, the boy took hold of one of her wrists and for no apparent reason twisted it until she almost cried out in pain. She insisted he did not seem to wish to hurt her and was very contrite afterwards. She asked with anxious tears what the incident meant, admitting that she felt helpless about how to deal with it and that she had permitted the child to hurt her. Discussion of the incident led to further clarification of her deep pleasure in her martyr-like submission to his whims and her smothering impulses towards him, her disgust with this in herself, and her consequent fear that either the child or she herself or both were in some way "abnormal."

It is both unnecessary and too early to report in detail the changes already evident in the boy's behavior and attitudes after about six months' separation from his mother and exposure to a human atmosphere of greater consistent firmness and security, which deprives him of any gain from his provocativeness but permits him to gain approval and satisfaction for acceptable behavior. It will suffice to say that the teachers report a progressive increase in his attention span, slowly growing interest in school work, decrease of erratic, destructive, distractible hyperactivity, and more consistent concern about the rights of others, both adults and his schoolmates. It is the distinct impression of the school psychologist that he has at least average intelligence and that prognosis for further improvement in his personality disorder is good if the mother's anxieties can be sufficiently relieved to prevent premature interruption of the régime.[3]

DISCUSSION

From studies such as the one detailed above, it seems to me that certain conclusions are possible. First, there is little to be gained from considering the energizing sources of human behavior from

---

[3]Unfortunately, follow-up data on this boy is not available. The therapist had to leave for military service at this point in the treatment, and upon discharge did not return to the same clinic.

the point of view of one or two instincts. Biologically, the human organism may be characterized as possessing a given set of inherited potentialities for growth and learning, and certain basic needs (4,10). These differ in degree from person to person and appear at somewhat different times in the life cycle. Universal to all human beings, however, are the needs of hunger, sex, and protection during relatively helpless periods of life. Possessing such needs and the given potentialities for acquiring mastery of techniques to satisfy them, either more or less independently or with other persons, the human being is subjected from the moment of birth to disciplines which are either directive and permissive, or limiting and prohibitive. It is important to recognize that it makes little difference so far as the results of this interaction are concerned whether these disciplines are applied consciously or unconsciously by the disciplinarians. It makes a great deal of difference whether those same disciplinarians (or others sharing their limitations of awareness of effective interpersonal realities) will or will not regard the errant behavior of offspring with pained surprise, feelings of injured innocence, and the baffled attitude of a hen watching ducklings—over which she has so patiently brooded—take to water.

The attitude toward the self which we call "security," "self-confidence," or "aggressive initiative" is, of course, relative to a particular situation which a person may face with his particular skills; but beyond these limits it is the result of a long series of previous experiences of success achieved with the approval or unconscious permissiveness of the authorities. If a particular behavior, having interpersonal significance and satisfying a need or drive, has thus been integrated with the full conscious approval of the parent or his surrogates, the person will feel neither guilt nor anxiety, nor will he show any lack of integration in this activity. If, on the other hand, a particular behavioral tendency has met with only unconscious and often guilty permissiveness on the part of the disciplinarian, the person so treated eventually may be more or less unable to inhibit that activity or give a coherently rational explanation of it, and may feel anxiety, guilt, or regret only after the act, or at the imminent displeasure of others concerned. A similar result occurs when a particular behavior—whether erotic, sexual, excessively dependent, demanding, or hostile—has been subjected to prohibitive discipline without sufficient reward for compliance to the discipline. The combination of firm prohibition coupled with adequate reward for submission is essential for experiences which after sufficient training lead to secure dissociation of particular impulses from the self-organization and to development within the self of feelings of repugnance, shame, or guilt with regard to them.

Under circumstances in which a person has not been allowed or even encouraged to develop other techniques for satisfaction of particular needs, one regularly observes varying degrees of defiant indulgence in forbidden activities, or self-gratification at opportune moments. Such indulgence may be followed by varying degrees of genuine guilt or perhaps only by lip-service to the culturally acceptable attitude toward the proscribed behavior by rationalization, or by fantastic distortions of one's own or the other's attitudes.

Clinical experience with children whose behavior is primarily a problem to others, and concurrent therapeutic effort with the parent, leaves the impression that the genesis of some of the characteristics of the psychopathic personality is no greater mystery than is that of other syndromes in psychopathology. Almost literally, in no instance in which adequate psychiatric therapeutic study of both parent and child has been possible has it been difficult to obtain sufficient evidence to reconstruct the chief dynamics in the ontogeny of the situation (3).[4] Regularly the more important parent—usually the mother, although the father is very often in some way involved—has been seen unconsciously to encourage the amoral or antisocial behavior of the child. The neurotic needs of the parent, whether of excessively dominating, dependent, or erotic character, are vicariously gratified by the behavior of the child, or in relation to the child. Such neurotic needs of the parent exist either because of an inability to satisfy them in the world of adults, or because of stunting experiences in the parent's own childhood— or more commonly, because of a combination of both of these factors. Because these parental needs are unintegrated, unconscious, and unacceptable to the parent himself, the child in every instance is sooner or later frustrated, and thus experiences no durable satisfactions. Because the indulgence or permissiveness of the parent in regard to marked overt hostility or to some mastery techniques, for example, is uncertain and inconsistent, control over the former or acquisition of the latter by the child is similarly uncertain and confused. If parental discipline is administered with guilt, it permits the child to exploit and subtly to blackmail the parent until the particular issue between them is befogged and piled high with irrelevant bickerings and implied or expressed mutual recriminations. When the parent's need for affection from the child is partly re-

---

[4]Collaborative treatment by two psychiatrists at this clinic of a series of children with school phobias has led to a still deeper insight into the close interdependence of emotional states of parent and child, and the advantages of concomitant therapy for relief of the difficulties in both. A report of this work has been published (3).

sponsible for alternating infantilization of the child and an extreme demand for unrealistic perfection, the situation is especially unpromising either for durable, adequate gratification of the child's actual dependent needs or for sufficient reward for such achievements as the child may attain.

The parent's selfish attempt to gain satisfaction for his urgent unconscious needs through the activity of the child leads to the various distortions of the child's self-regard and are expressed in the psychopathology of childhood. The child cannot gain full acceptance from the parent and hence from himself unless he achieves an impossible perfection. Thus greatly frustrated in his dependent needs when a child, he will when an adult, continually seek their gratification by fantasies, either verbalized or acted out with others, and never will be content with what he finds. In his extreme concern and uncertainty about himself, the child's behavior may include extremes of ingratiation. He may present such convincing distortions of his real attitudes toward himself and others that they frequently pass as a "sense of obligation" or of "love," and these distortions gratify for the moment the unconscious infantile wishes, and hence the illusions, of both parent and child. Since the implied promise of such bliss sooner or later becomes quite evidently impossible of fulfillment, the immature adult becomes either suddenly cold and impervious to social obligation or manifests an impotent fury carried out both on the other person and on himself, in some self-frustrating activity or symptom. In the rage at being "taken in," the "victim" of all these advances vacillates between doubting his own sanity and doubting that of the "psychopath." To the extent that he—the "victim"—is more thoroughly integrated, he perceives correctly the impermanence of the "psychopath's" enthusiasms and wonders whether the "psychopath" wasn't just "born that way."

REFERENCES

1. ALEXANDER, F. Neurotic character. Internat. J. Psychoanal., 11:292-311, 1930.

2. DUNN, W. The psychopath in the armed forces. Psychiatry, 3:251-259, 1941.

3. JOHNSON, A. M., FALSTEIN, E. I., SZUREK, S. A., and SVENDSEN, M. School phobia. Am. J. Orthopsychiat., 9:702-708, 1941. (Also in Learning and Its Disorders, The Langley Porter Child Psychiatry Series, Vol. 1. Palo Alto, Calif.: Science and Behavior Books, Inc., 1965.)

4. KARDINER, A. The individual and his society. New York: Columbia University Press, 1939.

5. MEAD, G. H. In C. W. Morris (Ed.) Mind, self, and society. Chicago: University of Chicago Press, 1934.

6. MENNINGER, K. A. Recognizing and renaming "psychopathic personalities." Bull. Menninger Clinic, 5:150-156, 1941.

7. PARTRIDGE, G. E. The psychopathic individual: A symposium. Mental Hygiene, 8:174-201, 1924.

8. PARTRIDGE, G. E. Current conceptions of psychopathic personality. Am. J. Psychiat., 10:53-99, 1930.

9. PRESTON, G. Psychiatry for the curious. New York: Farrar and Rinehart, 1940.

10. SULLIVAN, H. S. Conceptions of modern psychiatry. Psychiatry, 3:1-117, 1940.

THE GENESIS OF ANTISOCIAL ACTING-OUT IN CHILDREN AND ADULTS*

Adelaide M. Johnson and S. A. Szurek

The character problems we shall consider here are those of young children and adolescents in conflict with parents or some other external authority because of an acting-out of forbidden, antisocial impulses. There is no generalized weakness of the superego, but rather a superego defect in circumscribed areas of behavior. These defects may be termed "superego lacunae." For instance, a child may be entirely dependable in virtually every sphere of activity, regular in school attendance, and honest in his work, but he engages in petty stealing or perhaps in serious sexual acting-out. Mild to severe neurotic conflicts usually accompany such superego lacunae. We are not immediately concerned with the socially determined delinquency of slum children in which individual superego defects are not involved. Nor shall we discuss delinquent children reared in institutions, deprived of a sustained personal relationship, although some understanding of such children may be derived from our discussion.

The thesis is "that the parents may find vicarious gratification of their own poorly-integrated forbidden impulses in the acting out of the child, through their unconscious permissiveness or inconsistency toward the child in these spheres of behavior. The child's superego lacunae correspond to similar (unconscious) defects of the parents' superegos which in turn were derived from the conscious or unconscious permissiveness of their own parents" (9). These conclusions are the results of the collaborative study and treatment of the child and the significant parent or parents, as reported briefly by Szurek and Johnson (1,4,10,16).

---

*Reprinted with permission from The Psychoanalytic Quarterly, 21:323-343, 1952.

CONCEPTS OF DELINQUENCY

The literature contains a variety of descriptions and discussions of the etiology of circumscribed superego defects. Reich (14) coined the term "impulsive character." Alexander (2) conceived of the need for self-punishment as a motive for acting-out. Granted that these patients frequently suffer from neurotic guilt, the question remains why the resolution of guilt is sought specifically in acting-out.

Schmideberg (15) believed that people who act out their conflicts have a greater constitutional inability to tolerate frustration than more inhibited persons. Greenacre (7) reported in some detail a number of cases of psychopathic personality, but without concomitant study of the parents. She found that the fathers of such patients were usually ambitious and prominent, and the mothers usually frivolous and superficial, giving little attention to the home. She discussed the interrelationships of such parents with the child with respect to the child's superego development, but did not report defects in the parents' superegos.

Aichhorn (1) very early lent great impetus to investigations in this area. He, as well as Healy and Bronner (8), stated that some antisocial children have identified themselves with the gross ethical distortions of their parents. These observers noted such gross pathological correlations as forgery by the parent and stealing by the child, although they did not report the subtle unconscious correlations described here. Healy and Bronner attributed the child's inability to develop a normal superego to coldness and rejection by the parents, with the effect that one child in a family may steal while another will not, depending upon the one being unloved and the other loved. Other authors have stressed the patient's failure to receive sufficient love and warmth, so a strong positive identification with loving parents is impossible. Lack of love is considered by many to be the basic cause of superego defects. Even granting that unloved children may not develop a normal superego, it does not follow that coldness of parents alone can lead to the superego lacunae under discussion. Some very cold parents can create such great guilt or need to make restitution to a needed object that a very punitive superego is developed in the child. It is equally true that there are also relatively warm parents whose child may act out antisocially.

PARENTAL ATTITUDES

What constitutes "love" and "warmth" needs definition. If these include rationalization by a parent of guilt about his own sadomasochistic impulses, and appear as "gentleness" or "indulgence," the child experiences them as parental acceptance of his behavior. Firmness by the parents with respect to the form of expression of the child's egocentric or revengeful impulse is to be distinguished from sadistic suppression. Firmness bespeaks a parent who has learned how to gratify all his essential egocentric impulses non-destructively to himself and to others; such firmness may be devoid of masochistic or sadistic coloring and distortion. The stable parent has learned that his own interests eventually may be gratified in some measure, or he can choose which interest is preeminent, while clearly recognizing and accepting the consequences of his choice. He may even have learned how all of his major goals may be reached in some creative course of action. He may have the capacity to experiment before committing all his energies to any goal, and continue flexibly to search out the way to satisfaction of his major needs and wishes.

Such parental attitudes provide a child with various experiences encouraging him in turn to anticipate that his basic impulses eventually are gratifiable; that his disappointment, rage, or revengefulness at delays to his satisfactions are understood and accepted as natural reactions, but that their form of expression may invite retaliation from others; and finally, that the parent will patiently respect such reactive feelings, prolonged though they may be. In short, there are generally ways of obtaining sensual and other satisfactions at appropriate times and places, with appropriate people. Pertinent and amplified discussions of the concepts of "love," "guilt," and "restitution" have been presented elsewhere by Johnson (11).

STUDIES OF PARENT AND CHILD

In 1939, the authors and their colleagues (12,18) at the Institute for Juvenile Research of the University of Illinois, observed in their collaborative therapy studies of neurotic children and their parents that the parental neurosis often provided the unconscious impetus to the child's neurosis. It seemed logical, therefore, in the cases of the delinquents, to seek some possible links between the superego of parents and the child, even when the parents themselves were not known to act out. As a result of this work, Szurek (16) briefly described the psychopathic personality as a defect in personality organization, especially a defect in the individual's conscience, and he also defined its genesis. He clearly distinguished between the psychopathic personality and the delinquency of slum children, which is socially derived and does not involve individual superego defects. [See pages 3-5 of this book.]

Interestingly enough, Ferenczi (6) in an address on "Confusion of Tongues between the Adult and the Child" (read in 1932 but not published until 1949), arrived at a similar point of view. His sound concepts of the etiology of character and superego disturbances in children were based upon deductions from his experiences with the transference and countertransference of patient and analyst, rather than upon clinical evidence derived from the study of child and parent. Emch (4) explored similar concepts, independently and productively.

The unwitting employment of the child to act out for the parent his own poorly integrated and forbidden impulses was observed by us in parents of all economic and educational levels with the frequency, regularity, and predictability of a well-defined psychological mechanism determining human behavior.

SELECTION OF THE SCAPEGOAT

The subtle manner in which one child was unconsciously selected from several children as the scapegoat to act out for the parent was striking. Analytic study of the significant parent showed unmistakably the unique significance of this child to the parent, and the tragic pattern of parent and child moving inexorably, and usually unconsciously, in a fatal march of events. A profound sympathy was evoked for these consciously well-intentioned parents, whose unconscious needs were unwittingly inviting disaster upon the family.

A striking illustration of scapegoat selection occurred in several families whose children included an adopted child. The common pattern was parental acting-out through the adopted child, which conveniently provided the rationalization of inheritance to account for the child's delinquency. In other instances, parental guilt, born of unconscious hostility toward one child, made firmness and fair-dealing difficult. Parental vacillations appeared to be critical factors in the genesis of specific superego lacunae.

The sources of such hostility by the parent were varied. The child may have unconsciously become a rival for the indulgence of the other parent. The child may have represented a parent's sibling with whom the parent had unresolved sibling rivaly. The child may have been born or reared at times of high tension between parents. These and numerous other factors and combinations of factors contributed to parental hostility.

Frequently a dual purpose is served: not only is the parent's forbidden impulse acted out vicariously by the unfortunate child, but this very acting-out, in a manner distinctly foreign to the conscious wishes of the parent, provides a channel for the hostile, destructive impulses of the parent toward the child. Parents may blatantly reveal the child's acting-out to schools, family friends, and neighbors, in a way most destructive of the child's reputation, and this may become a source of great rage to the child. An adolescent girl recently hanged herself because her mother, missing ten dollars, telephoned the school authorities to have them search the girl's purse. In such cases the hostility of the parent is doubly directed: inwardly, toward the parent's own ego, and outwardly, toward the child.

Similarly, the child unknowingly exposes the parents to all degrees of suffering through his acting-out. One mother, revealing that her six-year-old daughter's constant masturbation at home and at school was a repetition of her own childhood experience, was frightened lest her husband learn of the latter. To observe her child flagrantly masturbating was thus doubly agonizing. The acting-out may often be an exaggerated portrayal of the unconscious impulses of the parent. Again, the child's hostility is doubly directed: toward his own ego as well as toward the egos of his parents.

EARLY SUPEREGO RIGIDITY

In order to recognize the evidence of destructive sanctions in less integrated parents, we must first understand the behavior of a well integrated parent, and the subtle conscious and unconscious ways in which his behavior directs the child's superego development. To be sure, the resolution of the oedipus conflict puts the definitive seal on the superego, but it is well to be aware of all the preoedipal and oedipal subtleties occurring in the family during this development. To the child in the early and middle latency period, there may be alternative modes of reacting on an ego level, but when the superego is involved the child normally is reared as if there could be no alternative reaction to the suppression of the impulses to theft, murder, truancy, and so on. The well-integrated, mature mother who tells a child to do something does not immediately check to see if it has been done, nor does she suggest beforehand that if it is not done there will be serious consequences.

Constant checking or warning often means to the child that there is an alternative to the mother's order and an alternate image of him in the mother's mind. Identification with the parent does not consist merely of identification with the manifest behavior of the parent. It necessarily includes a sharing by the child of the parent's conscious and unconscious concept of the child as one who is loved and honest, or sometimes unloved and dishonest. It is essential to appreciate this fact if we are to understand the etiology of superego defects and plan a rational therapy. Angry orders, suspiciousness, or commands colored by feelings of guilt convey to the child the doubtful alternative image of him in the parent's mind. The mature mother expects the thing to be done, and later if she finds the child has sidestepped her wishes, she insists, without guilt on her part, that it be done. The mother must have this firm, undoubting, unconscious assurance that her child will soon make her intention his own in accordance with her own image of him. This, however, produces a rather rigid and inflexible attitude in the young child. According to Fenichel (5), "After the dissolution of the oedipus complex . . . the superego is at first rigid and strict . . . and . . . later in normal persons it becomes more amenable to the ego, more plastic and more sensible."

In adolescence the superego normally is still fairly rigid, and the child is greatly disturbed when adults express doubts about his probity. Nothing angers adolescents more than to be warned about, or accused of, indiscretions of which they are not guilty. Such lack of faith in them threatens their repressive defenses, lowers their self-esteem, and weakens their assurance that they will do what is right. It suggests an alternative code of behavior which at that age frightens them.

Let us examine the evidence for the hypotheses developed, as revealed in some relatively uncomplicated cases of superego lacunae, although still recognizing that a child may evolve and employ character defenses constructed from multiple determinants.

Truancy. How does truancy originate? Parental coldness and rejection are insufficient causes, contrary to some authors; these are non-specific stimuli. The child of six, sensing coldness and rejection, may say angrily: "You don't love me—nobody loves me—I hate you all!" Then, and not infrequently, the specific stimulus may be applied by the parent: "Very well! Why don't you just pack your bag and go live some place else if you think we're so awful?" We have observed that some parents even go so far as to pack the child's suitcase—a terrifying experience for the child. The suggestion to "run away" comes more frequently from inside the home than outside, for rarely do small children tell their friends that their parents are "mean," or get suggestions from other children to leave home.

How an adult can initiate "running away" is found in an illuminating account by Aichhorn (1), who deliberately resorted to such provocation as a technique of treatment. In managing the transference, he purposely used a simple suggestive device to provoke a boy to run away from the institution. His aim was to establish a positive contact with the adolescent, in which he had been unsuccessful. This very narcissistic boy, with no positive feeling for Aichhorn, constantly complained about the institution. Aichhorn made subtle suggestions about the attractiveness of the outside world, and an

hour later the boy ran away, as Aichhorn had anticipated. In keeping with the therapist's predictions, some days later the boy returned, having found the outside world uninviting. He entered at
once into a positive relationship with Aichhorn.

Six-year-old Stevie is a good example of fulfilling a parent's
need for vicarious gratification. The child had been running away
since he was four. That his father knew an inordinate amount of
detail concerning the boy's episodes of exploration struck us as
very significant. This father reported that during these same two
years he himself had been forced to discontinue his work as driver
of a transcontinental truck, a job in which he had revelled. His
present job confined him to the city. It was striking to observe this
father asking Stevie to tell of his most recent escapade and, when
the child guiltily hesitated, supplying an intriguing reminder. The
account obviously fascinated the father, who eagerly prompted the
child from time to time. Then suddenly the father angrily interrupted the child with, "That's enough, Stevie; now do you see what
I mean, Doctor?" Stevie could not fail to sense his father's keen
interest and pleasure in his tale upon each return home, despite
the inevitable whipping. The father was a kind, well-intentioned
man who rightly feared for his little son's safety; but he was quite
unconscious of the fact that the stimulus of his own thwarted need
to travel was easily conveyed to the small, bright boy of whom the
father said: "Stevie's really a good kid—he would follow me around
the top of a wall fifty feet high." A smile of tacit but unwitting
approval often belies a parent's complaints about impulsive and
daring behavior by the child brought for treatment.

Helpless resignation in one area of the child's behavior and firm
conviction in another area are common among the parents under
consideration. On the one hand, effective action regarding a child's
temper tantrums may seem hopeless; on the other hand, there may
be unquestioned prohibition of the child's violence to a sibling or
the destruction of objects in the house.

Summarizing, we found that careful examination of parents and
children in cases of the children's running away revealed that it
was the parents who unconsciously provided the specific stimulus
for the defections, impelled by such motives as a need for vicarious gratification, or hostility, or both.

Stealing. Similar mechanisms operate in petty stealing by children. A woman patient, in analysis for nine months, became very
angry at her nine-year-old daughter, who was detected stealing
money from the teacher's desk. The patient stated that she knew
Margaret had occasionally taken nickels from her purse since she
was six or seven, but had said nothing, believing that Margaret
would "outgrow it"; besides, "it was never serious, so the less

said the better." The mature mother, we have observed, does not anticipate trouble or constantly check up on her child. But neither does she dismiss a significant transgression as unimportant; instead, she promptly resolves the problem without anxiety or guilt. She is neither the nagging, checking detective, nor the permissive, lax condoner.

During the same analytic hour, the patient recounted a recent dream, in which she stole a beautiful object from an elegant store. The therapist remarked upon the patient's failure to project the theft upon some other culprit. "Perhaps you are generally permissive of minor thefts?" For the first time the patient told of her own frequent stealing in childhood and adolescence; her mother had always protected her.

Three generations revealed themselves: our patient, after acquiring considerable insight, clearly recognized her own mother's countless little deceptions and covert permissiveness with the two grandchildren. Hitherto unnoticed, her mother's deviousness now carried meaning in the light of her own new understanding, and the grandmother's visits were curtailed until the grandchildren were older. As the analysis progressed, the patient was able to take a definite stand with her daughter, without anxiety or vacillation, without the permissiveness born of the need for vicarious gratification. The child stopped stealing. Formerly unhappy and unpopular, she became a favorite and outstanding pupil at school.

This mother's behavior reveals an attitude commonly observed in parents of children who steal. The parent whose own superego is defective will say, "My child will outgrow this fault." Often, it is the parent who is not involved in the acting out who finally insists upon treatment for the child. "He will outgrow it" is the permissive, protective attitude that keeps the problem active. At the first suggestion of criticism from outside the home, many such parents, whose own poorly integrated prohibitions permit them to overlook slight offenses, suddenly react with guilt and alarm, with righteous accusations and punishment of their child. The child is confused and angry at the parental betrayal. If he is not too ashamed or frightened, he may give voice to his recollections of similar parental deceptions, initiating a vicious cycle of hostile blackmail and mutual corruption.

Another illustration was seen in the adopted adolescent son of the head cashier in a large manufacturing concern. The son was brought for treatment because of stealing. The thefts were revealed when the mother surreptitiously secured (actually stole) the key to the boy's diary and discovered a well-ordered bookkeeping system of amounts extracted from guests' purses balanced against his own expenditures. The mother's duplicity was exceeded by that of the father, who, though scrupulously honest in business, had for two summers confiscated checks the boy received in payment for employment by the father's firm. To the boy, such behavior was not only an outrage but an obvious sanction for his own predatory behavior.

Many have observed that children and adults with severe compulsive neurotic symptoms, such as intensive handwashing, may also steal repeatedly. Such stealing, or the kleptomania of adults, again denotes the existence of one defect in the superego through which the patient may act out tension. Our detailed study of such stealing in adult patients with a compulsive neurosis shows clearly whence this permission stemmed.

There are many variations on the main theme that deception encourages deception, such as the admonition of the mother who says to the child: "Here is a dollar, but don't tell your father." To evaluate integrity as a virtue is difficult for a child who has repeatedly experienced broken promises, lightly made and disregarded without explanation or apology. The "more sensible" superego of the parent forgets the rigidity of the superego of the six- to nine-year-old to whom such behavior is not "sensible" but dishonest.

Perhaps the concepts in this section may best be epitomized by the words of a nine-year-old girl who asked the therapist, "When is my mother going to do her own stealing?"

Sexual Aberrations. Sexual aberrations also have become more understandable to us when viewed in the context of parent-child relationships. In several cases of long-standing overt homosexuality, search has revealed an unintentional fostering of some aberration by one of the parents. If this is true of patients in conflict and seeking treatment, one can but conjecture how great is the superego defect in cases in which the overt homosexuality arouses little or no conflict and no desire for treatment.

Little boys and girls in the oedipal or earlier stages may insist on being the opposite sex and wearing the clothes of the opposite sex. Detailed collaborative therapy in these cases has revealed a fostering influence by one parent, such as the mother who gave her six-year-old boy all her castoff clothes. Interestingly, the boy's desire to be a girl dated from the birth of a favored little sister three years earlier.

A young man of great professional talents had been an overt homosexual from the age of eighteen, at which time his mother told him that his father was not her husband. The mother's hostile motivation was clear. The youth's unconscious rage was the immediate, potent determinant of his homosexual turning to men as a protection against murdering a woman. The precipitating event occurred in a family setting, characterized by distorted adjustments and undue maternal permissiveness, which began in the patient's childhood. His rage at rejection by his real father was rapidly eroticized.

We have recently treated two men whose mothers were grossly maladjusted maritally and extravagantly seductive with their sons. The mother of one twenty-year-old said to him when his father was dying, "Jim, I'm madly in love with you; you are so handsome." This was but the culmination of years of varying degrees of seduction. The major factor in the patient's passive homosexuality had been the protection afforded by his father against murdering his mother, even transcending in importance his fear of his father, tremendous as it was. This young man refrained from overt homosexuality only with a great struggle, and came to analysis very disturbed.

A colleague of ours (13) treated a homosexual young man whose mother had the adolescent son escort her clandestine lovers home "to make things look better." The boy, aware of everything, eroticized his rage toward these men, spiting his mother as well.

The unconscious sanctions of parents, and their seductions of sons and daughters into homosexuality, are revealed by their guilty, anxious, or angry interrogations into the children's early conscious or unconscious homosexual play and explorations. Thereby may be stubbornly fixed what otherwise might have been a transient stage of normal growth. The heterosexual or homosexual acting-out of a child is thus parentally guided.

A depressed, forty-two-year-old woman came to consultation complaining primarily of the sadistic promiscuity of her twenty-year-old son. Since his adolescence, the mother had intently absorbed the minutest details of his accounts of intimacies with girls. The patient's husband was a beaten and submissive man. The sources of her ambivalent seductiveness with her son were easily adduced. Her own father was a Don Juan. From her early adolescence he came to her bedroom nightly to fondle her and even made attempts to enter her bed. At the first such instance, the patient sought protection from her mother. But the mother did not dare reproach the father, "lest he kill her." From the father, to the patient, to her son, sanctions of the forbidden are evident in three generations. The son, refusing treatment, will provide still another generation toward the biblical ten.

Among adolescents whose parents we also have been able to study we have seen no exhibitionism or voyeurism that has not revealed indubitably from which parent the necessary sanction stemmed. Admittedly, the opportunity to study such parents is limited; they refuse or soon discontinue treatment. The neurotic conflicts that contribute to exhibitionism and voyeurism are undoubtedly multiply-determined, but we have been concerned here only with the immediate mechanism which precipitates acting-out.

SANCTIONS FOR ACTING-OUT

The fantasies, hopes, and fears expressed by parents regarding some behavior of a child are a common and powerful influence toward healthy or maladapted living. Horrified parental anxiety over some behavior is expressed to the child: "You are beyond me; I can't handle you any more; if this doesn't stop, you will end in the reform school." Or, "You are just like your uncle; he came to a bad end." Parental fantasy guides the child's course of action.

Mothers who have seriously erred premaritally often betray acute anxiety regarding their daughters' behavior on dates. Accusations, detailed questioning, and dire warnings, rather than preventing undesirable behavior, constitute unwitting permissions. The overly anxious mother with poorly integrated promiscuous impulses or reaction-formations against sex may function similarly, even though she may never have acted out. The father also may contribute. Exasperating rigidity about dating, with a casual provocative suggestion, often upsets the balance. Only close collaboration between the two therapists of the parent and the child can reveal the unmistakable mutual provocation.

Early in analysis one mother glossed over an account of sexual acting-out as a girl, in which there had been no conscious fear of pregnancy. A year later in her analysis, anxiety developed lest her young daughter " . . . may go with a fast crowd, drink and get into trouble. All adolescent girls do too much sexual playing. One eggs on the other. I will worry about her getting pregnant. A girl cheapens herself. It's degrading. I don't know how to warn her but I must." The mother's poorly integrated masochistic impulses, partially repressed, were projected to the child. Not consciously fearful of pregnancy herself, she nevertheless feared her child's being cheapened and becoming pregnant. Her fantasies implied destructiveness to the child as well as vicarious gratification for her own repressed impulses. Eventually, the patient revealed that her stepmother, as glamorous as she was unstable, had frequently discussed sex and had suggested, "You will probably be more highly sexed than your stepsister—and have more trouble!" The stepmother subsequently had been entranced with lurid accounts of the patient's dates. The patient's analysis fortunately progressed so that the heritage from the stepmother was not transmitted to the daughter, whose dates no longer aroused undue anxiety.

In the parental voicing of fears for the imagined acts of a child—even of violence—the transmitted image of the act leaves a bolder imprint than the fear of it. An infant on the lap of a social worker colleague put his hands about her neck. With genuine fright, the mother said, "I hope my son won't be a killer!" By the age of fifteen, he was. Another mother, reading a news account of a brutal murder, said to her son, "I'm glad it wasn't you who did it." His crimes soon eclipsed those of the news story.

Analysts themselves must take care lest they inadvertently provide sanctions for acting-out by their patients, be they children or adults. Patients displaying sexual perversions or even more serious antisocial tendencies are sometimes warned that they may act out. Such a warning to a patient with a defective superego can be tragically destructive, ruining the developing structure of the patient's belief in the therapist's ethical concept of him. Warning or questioning without factual justification may be interpreted both as a humiliation and a permission.

We believe such warnings against acting-out are to be distinguished clearly from Freud's concept of warning the patient against future acting-out in the transference. To warn a patient regarding acting-out of the transference is entirely different from the warning against antisocial impulses outside the analytic hour. In fact, Freud warned analysts against too rapid mobilization and interpretation of impulses that might be dangerously expressed outside the analytic hour, particularly sadism. A loose and unclear concept of what is meant by "acting-out" has led a number of analysts to carry over Freud's suggestions about acting-out in the transference to the acting-out in a serious antisocial way.

COLLABORATIVE THERAPY

The concepts presented in this paper could not have been developed, nor could they have been subjected to further scrutiny, except by simultaneous study of parent and child. Such studies can be carried out by two collaborating therapists, if they are unambivalent, uncompetitive and entirely cooperative, or by a single skilled therapist experienced in collaborative therapy dealing with both parent and child.

Prior to our appreciation of this principle, we repeatedly failed to understand relatively simple cases of acting-out, despite frequent treatment periods (four to five hours per week) extended for months or years. Our consistent warmth and affection failed to stay the continued stealing, truancy, or sexual acting-out. It is now apparent that any guilt the child may have mustered toward us was readily dissolved by unconscious permissions at home. The child became increasingly confused and fearful of us, and resolved his immediate conflict by discontinuing treatment. Instances of acting-out were successfully managed only if we could either treat the significant parent or separate the child from parents during treatment. Treatment of the parent requires great care. If his role is unconscious, the uncovering of his own problems is a miserable ordeal for him. If the parent has provided conscious sanctions, treatment is usually impossible.

In serious acting-out, treatment of the child will be futile, and perhaps dangerous, unless the significant parent is also adequately treated or the child is separated from the home. The untreated parent can and does act out through the child, foisting responsibility upon the therapist, much as parents incriminate heredity for unacceptable behavior in adopted children.

We cannot here detail the therapeutic procedures employed. The broad outlines may be indicated and have been drawn in part in the preceding discussion.* Effective therapy necessitates the development of a positive and usually dependent attitude toward the therapist, with whom the patient may identify as an ego ideal. The patient first must be made guilty and neurotic in the area of his acting-out. The superego lacuna must be filled. In the process of arousing guilt with neuroticism about the previously unrestrained impulse, therapy continues. It culminates in analysis of the patient's conflicts. Ideally, the final result should be characterized by independence of the therapist; a consciously discriminating, reality-oriented ego function to supplant the superego lacuna; and a freedom from the former self-destructive, rebellious impulsiveness.

THE ROLE OF GUILT

Guilt, and a need for punishment, have been suggested by Alexander (3) and others as major etiological determinants of antisocial acting-out; they have cited as evidence the frequency with which such acts are rigged to facilitate detection. While examples are numerous, our experience has not borne out this concept of etiology. The sequence does not appear to be guilt, causing acting-out in order to be caught, thus assuaging guilt. Rather, it is unwitting parental prompting which causes acting-out, and it is our impression that the desire to be caught is a way of seeking protection against committing even worse offenses, which might incur extreme retaliation, even destruction.

The fear displayed by an apprehended delinquent child only simulates the genuine anxiety of an internalized conscience—neurotic

---

*For further discussion of therapy, see Searchlights on Delinquency, (9,17).

guilt. On the contrary, we have found that such fear frequently stems from anticipated punishment, with no guilt coloring.

In failing to appreciate this distinction, the analyst impressed with the apparent guilt of the offender may even foster further offenses by his immediate search for sources of unconscious guilt. There is unconscious guilt in abundance in the cases under discussion, as in all neurotic personalities. A welling tide of hostility against a young sibling may be effectively dammed by defenses. A crack in those defenses, created by unconscious parental permissiveness for a specific form of acting-out, may provide an outlet for the emotional energy. Thus, forbidden impulses, derived from a variety of neurotic conflicts, may find expression in stealing, arson, truancy, or worse, depending upon the nature of the sanctions. Very commonly, great guilt about sex is acted out in stealing, given appropriate parental permission.

These concepts indicate the error of probing for hidden guilt as the first approach to delinquents. With the crack in the defenses unsealed, the immediate result may be an increased impetus to act out, with even greater seriousness, through the permitted, though antisocial, channel. The first therapeutic efforts should be directed toward repairing the superego lacuna. In an adolescent who feels guilty about his hostility toward siblings and who unconsciously feels permitted to steal, unless the superego defect of stealing has been adequately managed, it is dangerous to mobilize the neurotic conflict with siblings, for the acting-out may then increase. Only later is it safe to proceed with a thorough analysis.

CONCLUSIONS

Science can seldom ascribe any phenomenon to a single cause. Our goal has been to emphasize a major cause of antisocial behavior while still recognizing that the antisocial child reared in a family is the product of a multiplicity of variables of mixed quality and quantity.

Scientific proof of causation is not satisfied by demonstrating the invariable presence of the suspected cause (unwitting parental permissiveness) whenever the effect (antisocial behavior of children) is observed. It must also be demonstrated that the suspected cause does not occur unless the effect is also seen. This, too, has been our experience. Parental permissions have never been revealed without ultimate antisocial behavior in at least one "scapegoat" child. The superego lacuna of the child has always been traceable to a specific parental permission. Our thesis is not post hoc ergo propter hoc: the enmeshing interplay of parent and child in the affected area bespeaks more than a fortuitous time sequence. Furthermore, we have observed that the outcome is doubly destructive toward the child's and the parent's ego organization, unless adequate therapy of both is provided.

REFERENCES

1. AICHHORN, A. Wayward youth. New York: Viking Press, 1935.
2. ALEXANDER, F. The neurotic character. Int. J. Psychoanal. 11:292-311, 1930.
3. ALEXANDER, F., et al. Psychoanalytic therapy: Principles and application. New York: Ronald, 1946.
4. EMCH, M. On "the need to know" as related to identification and acting out. Int. J. Psychoanal. 25:13-19, 1944.
5. FENICHEL, O. The psychoanalytic theory of neurosis. New York: W. W. Norton, 1945.
6. FERENCZI, S. Confusion of tongues between the adult and the child. Int. J. Psychoanal. 30:225-230, 1949.
7. GREENACRE, P. Conscience in the psychopath. Amer. J. Orthopsychiat. 15:495-509, 1945.
8. HEALY, W. & BRONNER, A. New light on delinquency and its treatment. Inst. of Human Relations Publ. New Haven: Yale University Press, 1936.
9. JOHNSON, A. M. Sanctions for superego lacunae of adolescents. In K. R. Eissler (Ed.), Searchlights on delinquency. New York: International Universities Press, 1949.
10. JOHNSON, A. M. Sanctions for superego lacunae. Paper read before the Chicago Psychoanalytic Society, March 25, 1947.
11. JOHNSON, A. M. Some etiologic aspects of repression, guilt, and hostility. This Quarterly. 20:511-527, 1951.
12. JOHNSON, A. M., FALSTEIN, E. I., SZUREK, S. A., & SVENDSEN, M. School phobia. Amer. J. Orthopsychiat. 11:702-711, 1941. Reprinted in I. N. Berlin & S. A. Szurek (Eds.), Learning and its disorders. Vol. 1, the Langley Porter Child Psychiatry Series. Palo Alto, Calif.: Science and Behavior Books, 1965.
13. KOLB, L. C. Personal communication.
14. REICH, W. Der triebhafte Charakter. Int. Psychoanal. Verlag, Vienna, 1925.
15. SCHMIDEBERG, M. The mode of operation of psychoanalytic therapy. Int. J. Psychoanal. 19:310-320, 1938.
16. SZUREK, S. A. Notes on the genesis of psychopathic personality trends. Psychiatry 5:1-6, 1942. (See page 3 of this volume.)

17. SZUREK, S. A. Some impressions from clinical experience with delinquents. In K. R. Eissler (Ed.), Searchlights on delinquency. New York: International Universities Press, 1949. (See page 72 of this volume.)

18. SZUREK, S. A., JOHNSON, A. M., & FALSTEIN, E. I. Collaborative psychiatric treatment of parent-child problems. Amer. J. Orthopsychiat. 12:511-516, 1942. Reprinted in S. A. Szurek & I. N. Berlin (Eds.), Training in therapeutic work with children. Vol. 2, the Langley Porter Child Psychiatry Series. Palo Alto, Calif.: Science and Behavior Books, 1967.

CONCERNING THE SEXUAL DISORDERS
OF PARENTS AND THEIR CHILDREN*

S. A. Szurek

Anyone who has had experience in psychiatric clinics for children knows the broad variety of impulsive behavior these young patients present, in both sexual and apparently nonsexual acts. Anyone who makes it a regular practice to interview an impulsive child's parents becomes aware of some connections between the child's behavior and the attitudes and behavior of his parents. Therapists working with impulsive children, who for practical and theoretical reasons regularly include concomitant therapeutic efforts with both parents, are becoming more and more convinced of an ever-present, intimately etiological, connection (2,4,8-14,16). One day a more complete chapter will be written based on therapeutic studies of families. That chapter will detail the connections which span the whole range of the psychopathological spectrum: from impulsive disorders through the neurotic illnesses to the psychoses (5,17,19,20,22). Some, like Dr. Adelaide Johnson and her coworkers (3), already have a wealth of clinical experience, only a portion of which is recorded in the literature. More of it is being "recorded" in the training experience of young psychiatrists who are learning to work with parents as well as with the child. This is perhaps more generally true in psychiatric clinics for children, but it occurs also in other centers where analyst-teachers bring to their teaching a background of working with parents of child patients.

There are good reasons for this paucity of literature. To work therapeutically with three people rather than with one requires time, often collaborators, as well as clarification of technical therapeutic principles and procedures deduced from these principles. Collaborators of equal training and sufficient sympathy to the idea not to allow ambivalences to cloud their vision of the im-

---

*Reprinted with permission from The Journal of Nervous & Mental Disease, 120:369-378, 1954.

port of clinical data so obtained are difficult to find and to keep working together in the same therapeutic community. Often it is necessary to train a team, which takes many years (18). Results of the team's work may not be, and in some respects cannot be, regarded as wholly and strictly comparable to clinical data obtained by the classical psychoanalytic method. Often these teams work in clinics, where analytic sessions are infrequent, and where elementary psychotherapeutic procedures have to be learned and taught to a constant stream of psychiatric trainees.

Nonetheless, it would be an error wholly to disregard clinical data and results obtained under these circumstances. Although frequency of therapeutic sessions may be low, the combination of prolonged therapy and the therapeutic skill of the more experienced members of these teams may partially compensate for whatever deficiency there may be in such work, as compared to psychoanalysis by formally trained, highly experienced analysts. The life history of the child is carefully compiled and correlated with the more readily recollectable events of the total family history and of the antemarital history of each parent. This compilation makes available the facts of the child's actual experience, especially in the first two or three years of life, and is a more reliable source of data than reconstructions based on information obtained in analysis. The contrast between the unconscious intrapsychic elaboration and/or distortion by the child of these events, and of the thus known actual attitudes of his parents, is then more apparent and more firmly grounded in empirical observation. The individual work of each member of the family with one or several therapists, frequently reviewed and collated with the observed effects (not only upon the patient's behavior but upon that of other members of his family), offers the therapeutic team an operational check of hypotheses that is in some measure comparable with the classical psychoanalytic method (1,21).

In brief, when the transferences of each parent and the child begin to be loosened in such therapeutic work, the release of even small amounts of energy from internalized conflicts in any one member of the family often results in potentiating effects within the family which at times offers dramatic validation of the postulated relations of symptom-formation or exacerbation in all three—child, mother, and father. This does not mean that therapeutic work, especially in the more severe disorders, can be shortened for thorough resolution of conflicts. It often does mean that simultaneous therapy with all three tends to reduce the more durable destructive effects of intercurrent crises on the personality development of the child. Now and then, it permits not only the reduction of on-going neurotic fixations, but also the reversal of the neurotic processes when therapeutic efforts with one member of the family either have failed or have proved insufficient to the task (3,22).

For these, and other reasons which cannot be discussed because of limitations of space, we turn to consideration of some clinical data derived from what is usually known as "psychotherapy," as distinct from "psychoanalysis," which may be of interest to both child-oriented and adult-oriented psychoanalysts.

CLINICAL ILLUSTRATIONS

An example of one type of sexual problem may be sketched very briefly from the staff's clinical data derived from nine months' experience with a fifteen-year-old girl and both of her parents.[1] A very anxious mother brought the second of her five children to the clinic, five or six days after severe phobias about going to school, death, and leaving her mother developed in the daughter. Therapeutic work with mother, daughter, and father, each being seen once a week by the same therapist, began about a month later, after several exploratory interviews. These interviews revealed decreasing family income, the father's premature ejaculations, the mother's lack of orgasm, and much quarreling between them. The daughter, who felt herself uglier than, less intelligent than, and envious of her seventeen-year-old sister, had begun secretly to have sexual relations with a boy four years her senior who was a "big wheel" in school. She experienced no orgasm with him but did obtain a great sense of pride and power; at the same time she felt extremely guilty about her sexual activity, her provocativeness, and was fearful that only her compliance with the boy's sexual demands would keep him interested in her. She hated her father, who had once told her that her mother had been sexually promiscuous and "no good" before their marriage. Although her initial phobias centered around staying near her mother and preventing the mother's leaving home without her, later her phobic symptoms spread and involved the whole family. She refused to go to movies and prevented, on occasion, the rest of the family from going by brandishing a knife, which made her father anxiously decide not to leave her home alone. He was afraid she might hurt someone, or herself, in her rage, which was what he himself feared _he_ would do when he became destructive in his own rages. One night the father found his daughter turning on the gas in the kitchen. She also was unable to sleep at night without a light during this period.

The mother, who frankly discussed her sexual dissatisfaction with her husband in her sessions, eventually revealed an extra-

---

[1] I am indebted to Robert Dalton, Ph.D., for the report of his work with this family.

marital affair about which she felt guilty, although it had been
sexually very satisfying. This affair had occurred sixteen years
earlier, just before she became pregnant with this daughter. The
mother felt extremely anxious and guilty about what part she might
have contributed to her daughter's illness. She also felt guilty
about her indulgence in phantasies concerning sexual affairs with
other men, even during coitus with her husband, and was afraid the
therapist would tell her husband of these phantasies. She deprecated
her husband, calling him a rabbit, saying his short stature made it
impossible for her to become sexually excited by him.

His size, she said, made her feel as if she were in bed with her
little brother. She had promised herself, when single, that she
would never marry a small man, and yet here she was tied to just
such a man. She compared her husband unfavorably to the therapist who, she felt, was better looking and more considerate of her
feelings. Incidentally, the daughter's phobias erupted in severe
form during the weekend of a visit by the mother's brother, although
the girl's sexual activity had been going on for the previous four
months, and she had been moderately anxious.

The father, lonely, rather isolated, and self-deprecatory all his
life, had lost both parents by death when he was five. He had felt
exploited by an older half-brother and his wife, on whose ranch he
worked until he ran away when he was eleven years old. After
several years of "knocking around," he got a job at a grocery store
where he worked for fifteen years. When the store closed, he became similarly steady in a post office job. He spoke of himself as
being always "very independent, maybe too much so." He was fearful of any close or tender feelings, recalling how a man he considered his friend once stole all his belongings in the middle of the
night. He was easily hurt and angered, as well as helplessly baffled, by the daughter's symptoms and the mother's neurotic involvement with her. When angry with his wife, he frequently did not come
home for meals, or slept in the afternoons at home. According to
the mother, he was generally uninterested in the four older children,
all of whom were girls, caring only for his youngest child, a boy.

The patient's school phobia abated six weeks after initiation of
therapy, shortly after her therapist discussed with her his understanding of her feelings but pointed out that it would be futile to
continue therapy unless she became actively concerned both with
her phobias and her sexual activity. During the week following this
interview, the mother went to church despite the daughter's protest,
and later the girl became more disturbed and confessed her affair
to her mother. The mother, smiling and occasionally laughing
while telling the therapist of the incident, "I didn't say anything for
two or three minutes, just walked up and down the floor trying to

decide what my reaction should be." Nevertheless, she told the father when he came home. When their daughter told them she had confided her affair to a cousin, both parents became very angry and slapped the girl, because she had not kept her sexual behavior a secret within the family.

Shortly thereafter, the girl stopped having coitus (although continuing some sexual play) with the boy, and very gradually during the next five months most of the phobias were reduced as daughter, mother, and father continued to work with the therapist until his departure from the staff. Both mother and daughter manifested strongly positive transference attitudes, at times competitive with each other, with the mother speaking frankly of her sexual feelings for the male therapist. The father, although suspicious that his wife—who looked better, gained weight, and lost many of her anxieties—was in love with some man, continued his work with the therapist with a generally positive attitude and gradually gained more confidence in himself.

There were repeated quarrels between the parents during this phase of therapy. These quarrels, however, tended to clarify the situation between them, unlike those prior to therapy, which ended in prolonged self-deprecation and sulky, hurt emotional isolation on the parts of both. The father told the mother several times in these later quarrels that she was free to seek a divorce; that she was as crazy as the daughter, whom she babied too much. At the same time the father became more aware of the effect, on himself and his family, of his previous prolonged periods of emotional estrangement; and although he stayed away from the holiday meals because of the mother's refusal to visit his relatives, he provided the money for the family's holiday.

The mother, accusing herself of being crazy for staying with her husband, became angry not only with her husband but with her daughter as well, and would leave home in the car for several hours. She became annoyed and irritated when her daughter refused to go for a ride with the family, in order to go out with her boyfriend, but "took out" her irritability on her husband. She gradually became aware of this and eventually recognized that in spite of his faults and her sexual dissatisfaction with him, she needed to stay with him because of the children, and that he was a good man who did the best he could, as did she herself. The mother, having decided to go back to work the following year, as she had done during the war, looked forward to this prospect both for the pleasure it would give her to be with other people, and for the relief it would offer for the family's financial problem. Both parents agreed to let the daughter decide whether she wished to go on in school or not, rather than—as mother had at first thought of doing—demanding that she stay at home and care for the youngest children while the mother worked.

An adolescent girl who came to our clinical attention when she was fourteen years old provides another clinical example. The following biographical sketch has been summarized from the statements of her parents.

The father, aged forty-two, a professional man, was seen only once at the clinic, when he gave information chiefly about the daughter and his life with her and the girl's mother, to whom he had never been formally married. The few other facts about him were obtained by other clinicians prior to the family's referral to the clinic. He was said to be the only child of European-born parents. He had his preprofessional education in Europe, and was said "not to believe in marriage." He was also described by the mother as artistic, Bohemian in tastes, irresponsible, but charming. At nineteen he was having affairs with many women while living openly with one, by whom he had two children. He left this woman to live with our patient's mother.

The attractive mother, aged 38, was separated from her third husband at the time of referral to the clinic. She was the only child of a sea captain and a woman to whom she remained closely attached most of her life. She feared that her daughter had inherited from herself and her father something "which should not be perpetuated," and she was determined never to have another child because it brought such frightening responsibilities. She saw the same problems in her husband's other illegitimate children. Although very concerned for her daughter, the mother was not really interested in any help for herself and, she said with hostility, came for interviews only because of the requirement of the juvenile court.

The parents had lived together until the daughter was about one and one-half years old. Thereafter, "because of temperamental differences," they were separated more often than they lived together until the child was six, when the separation was final; the father thereafter provided no financial support. The patient, when five years old, frequently "snuggled up and burrowed into adults," in a way that her father thought was more than "childish affectionateness." After leaving the father, the mother took the daughter to her own mother's home town for the next two and one-half years, sending her to a boarding school during the week. When the girl was eight, male neighbors complained to the mother that her daughter was too provocative with them in their homes, and asked the mother not to permit her to visit. When the mother confronted her with these complaints, the girl accused the neighbors of sexually approaching her. However, she also hugged and kissed several of her mother's boyfriends so effusively that some of them never returned. At the same time, the girl gave the impression of being very jealous of the relation between her mother and grandmother.

When the patient was eight and one-half, her mother lived and worked in the same city as her father, and she was sent to live with him, his third common-law wife, and their three children. The third wife was said to be an alcoholic who on a spree was arrested for neglect of the children. Our patient however, was so unruly that after one month her father returned her to her mother, who then experienced persistent difficulty with her because of her continued sexual interests and talk of sex with various people in the neighborhood. Having returned to the grandmother's city, the daughter was placed in two more boarding schools, each of which, in turn, refused to readmit her because of her tantrums, sexual interests, "dirty jokes," and bad influence upon the other pupils. When she was eleven years of age she lived with her father for four months, during which time she paraded in the nude before her seventy-three-year-old grandfather, whose young wife then left him. She was so sexually provocative with a married Japanese male house servant that he left, and she had violent temper tantrums when her father made futile efforts to keep her at home during the evenings. She accused her father of being sexually promiscuous, and she herself became obese and unclean.

About this time the mother married an orchestra leader and took the girl back, but again placed her in boarding school. At school, and also on weekends at home, her behavior became even more difficult. She sneaked out of windows at night to meet boys, or invited them into the house when her parents were away, using her allowance to buy them liquor. She later boasted of having had her first coitus at twelve with a man twice her age. When taken to a therapist, who gave a poor prognosis, she told him that her mother and grandmother performed cunnilingus upon her. She was placed in the Home of the Good Shepherd for several months, again told what were considered fantastic lies, and was the center of troublesome groups. The mother removed her, against advice, after her third husband left the country, and placed the girl in another boarding school, where she told other girls she was pregnant and needed an abortion.

After the school refused to readmit her for the next term, the mother in desperation returned the patient to her father, who was reluctant to take her again because of a recent coronary attack, and because he was separated from his third common-law wife. The girl was out most evenings, and talked of being pregnant. She said the father of the "child" could have been any one of thirty or forty men, either black or white, although upon examination she was found not to be pregnant. Three or four months later, she ran away from her father's home, phoned him repeatedly for money, telling him that she was in Mexico (and other places) and intended to marry a gangster. After her father's repeated requests, she returned home, saying that the gangster had given himself up. In a week or two she left home again; however, this time her father reported her disappearance to the police, who picked her up at an apartment where, she boasted, she had "taken on six or more teenage boys in a gang-bang on a dare."

While confined at the Juvenile Court detention home, the patient accused her father of having one of his female friends perform cunnilingus upon her, then of having a male friend have intercourse with her, and finally of the father himself having intercourse with her. She also said she had been raped by an abortionist, after she had had the benefit of his services. She eagerly looked forward to the front page publicity she would receive as a result of her father's trial.

Incidentally, the girl's mother sympathized with the father and testified in his defense. The girl rather boastfully repeated the stories of incest, cunnilingus, and intercourse to the court, and later to any clinician involved in the study of her problems. She did not know how she felt about "George," as she called her father, but said that he was quick-tempered and generally irascible. She claimed that her mother had had her only to hold her father, but she (the mother) should have known better since he had already left another woman to live with her. She "knew" her mother hated her, and she herself needed love since she had never experienced it. The various examiners commented on her apparent lack of guilt or anxiety.

At the Juvenile Court's insistence, the mother and daughter came to the clinic for weekly interviews, and were seen by rather young and inexperienced therapists for about three months, while the patient was kept in a closed home for girls. The father was not included in this work because he lived in a distant city, and was planning a trip to Europe after being exonerated of his daughter's accusations at his trial.

Throughout this period the mother continued to be deprecatory of herself, of the Juvenile Court authorities, and of the therapists. On the one hand, she was reluctant and anxious about again assuming parental responsibility for this girl, which she felt would almost entirely preclude earning her own living or having a life of her own. On the other hand, she guiltily wished to find someone else, medical or juvenile court authorities, to relieve her of any further responsibility for her daughter. By these attitudes she reflected her own deep doubts of her worth, lovability, and competence to take care of herself. At times she experienced a desperate need for a father surrogate, yet she feared she would again exploit and devour him, or be exploited and devoured by him. In her interviews, the intelligent, somewhat obese patient talked of having no faith in anything but wishing she did. She told of her confused feelings, of her need for love, and of her greater ease with older people than with persons nearer her own age. Her sophisticated manner, her expressed interest in art and dramatics, and her ambition to know prominent people covered an insatiable infantile yearning for passive gratifications at which she thus indirectly hinted. In the therapeutic situation, strong negative reactions were frequent following her therapist's refusal to convert the interviews into social discussions.

Both mother and daughter declined to continue with the successors to their first therapists, as the girl's behavior had become calmer and the probation officer's anxiety and concern were relieved. Consequently, the court's requirement of "forced psychotherapy" was removed when the girl and her mother agreed to live together again. A few months later, it was learned that the mother had been relieved of her responsibilities by the daughter's marriage to a man in his twenties, who was reportedly very fond of her. The mother was free to seek a fourth marriage partner.

A similar story of life-long impulsiveness, culminating in repeated attacks upon women in the streets, could be detailed about the adolescent son of a rather egocentric divorced couple who came to our clinic. The boy had been shunted between them over many years. The father was an impulsive person, repeatedly changed his work, residence, and women friends, of whom he made no secret to the boy. He even tried to provide the boy with sexual satisfaction at houses of prostitution as his unsuccessful attempts to cure his son of the penchant for knocking women down and as a result being arrested by the police.

The mother, an extremely neurotic woman with recurrent hysterical symptoms, sought and obtained the boy's release from the reformatory. She did this in part to get state financial assistance for his care, when she felt unable to continue her work as a sales clerk after a physician advised colpoplasty for an injury sustained during her son's birth. Her helplessness during a sudden hysterical attack of paralysis one evening led her, after lying on the floor all night, to ask her son in the morning to lift her back into bed. Although she appeared extremely guilty and anxious while telling her therapist about this, she continued to have the boy carry her back and forth from bed to the bathroom for several days. Not too long after this incident, the boy again was suspected by the police of several attacks upon women in the streets, though the charges were not confirmed.

Therapeutic work with the son and both parents was irregular and repeatedly interrupted, first by the father, who was very reluctant to assume any financial obligation for the boy, and later by the boy's own failure to keep his appointments regularly. Therapy ended after thirty months, when the boy was caught by the husband of a provocative young woman, whom he was coming to visit for the second time. He had followed her home from a movie on the previous evening and had been admitted, somewhat reluctantly, through a window, while the husband was away from home. The boy was eventually committed to the state hospital for the criminally insane for institutional study of his sexual aberration.

A fourth clinical experience, illustrative of yet another variety of impulsive sexual behavior, might exemplify—if space permitted a more detailed presentation—the dual factors of family history and current events in the family, which generate symptomatic behavior in a child.

A mother, a former nurse, brought her fourteen-year-old daughter to the clinic complaining that for more than three years the daughter had been extremely preoccupied with sex. She grabbed at her mother's breasts and struck them whenever her mother walked by. When angry—which was frequent—she pulled at her brother's or father's penis, and once kicked her father in the groin. This behavior had first appeared when she exposed her genitals to her brother, of whom she had always been jealous, later saying she wished to impress him with her pubic hair. Although she and a girlfriend had once done a strip act in front of a window at home, most of her exhibitionistic behavior was confined to the home. She was usually rather shy, withdrawn, and had few friends at school or in the neighborhood. Her mother said that she had feared the possibility of homosexual tendencies, because her daughter had frequently rubbed up against her breasts "in a very sexy way."

Upon investigation, it was learned that the mother herself had had repeated attacks of neurotic illness since her marriage, with which she was continually dissatisfied both sexually and financially. She had sought and received pediatric care for her daughter from the age of four, and almost continuous psychiatric service from the age of six. Early in the girl's childhood the mother was anxious about her daughter's masturbation, which began at two and one-half years of age, and asked pediatricians for repeated vaginal and urinary examinations, which were always negative for infection or other disease. Later, the mother complained on various occasions of her daughter's negativism, temper tantrums (which mother felt helpless to deal with), daydreaming, attacks of choreiform movements, sleeping poorly, doing poorly in school, and of being teased and abused by other children. Family service agencies, every psychiatric clinic in the city and several pediatricians knew of her, as the mother went from one clinic to another whenever she was discontented. Five months before her application to our clinic, the daughter had for ten days been in the psychopathic ward of the county hospital, where for a time she was considered as possibly schizophrenic. Her mother, too, was thought by various clinicians to be a "simple schizophrenic," "paranoid," or "untreatable." On one occasion her father had become very disturbed, thrown things, and experienced severe headaches, and her mother feared he would kill the family. Unfortunately, he was seen only once at a psychiatric clinic.

Closer scrutiny revealed that during the previous eleven years, each episode of the mother's increased complaints about her daughter was related to some event in the mother's or the family's life that was disturbing to the mother. Some of these events were: the murder of her brother, who was stabbed by the wife he had left; the father's loss of a job during the depression and the family's going on relief; the maternal grandmother's coming to live with the family and interfering with the parents' management of the children and with the mother's ability to experience orgasm in coitus while her mother was sleeping near their bedroom; the grandmother's subsequent sudden death from a skull fracture due to a fall down a flight of stairs while visiting her sister; the father's night work at one period; the mother's difficulty in learning welding during the war and her suspicion that her fellow students made unfavorable remarks about her; the father's reported periodically lessened sexual desire while the mother's libido increased; and subsequently, repeated staff changes in a psychiatric clinic she attended periodically and the staff's decreasing hopefulness about the outcome of their work with the mother.

Both mother and daughter were seen in regular interviews over a four-year period by a series of therapists, each of whom worked with one of them for at least a year. During this time many of the girl's original symptoms decreased markedly, and she did better in school, eventually graduating from high school. The mother became progressively less anxious and began to work again as a nurse during the last year of their visits to the clinic. It is not possible to do more than mention that, as the mother's neurotic anxieties and inhibitions about her own sexual impulses, about her rage, and about work were gradually reduced, similar problems of the daughter were also somewhat relieved in therapy, and the close neurotic nexus between them was loosened. Each then began to be able to have more satisfying relations with others, both within and outside of the family. These changes included both a lessening of the mother's sadomasochistic libidinous drive and a more consistent satisfaction in coitus.

Boys Who Murder

If space permitted, one could give similar vignettes of clinical experience with adolescent and preadolescent boys who have murdered girls. In those boys of whom we have any detailed knowledge, there appeared to be present an almost complete inhibition or denial of sexual impulses and interests. Generally, we could also discern some unconscious sexual provocation, or at least opportunities for sexual stimulation, of the boys by the mothers. Some of these mothers manifested severe repression of their own sexual and hostile impulses and a markedly immature, anxious helplessness about injuries which either they themselves or their sons had suffered. The sons recalled these episodes of injury and their mother's paralysis about taking care of them, with bitter, cold hostility and contempt. The father was either absent by death or was unassertive in the home in relation to the mother, and was sometimes sexually unfaithful to her.

Sexual Symptoms in Schizophrenic Children

We have also seen sadomasochistic sexual impulsiveness, or at least symptoms related to the genitalia, in several schizophrenic children. One boy's psychotic episode of about three years' duration began when he was four and one-half years old, after the birth of his only sister. During his hospitalization we saw, among other symptoms, prolonged efforts at tearing off his penis and an expressed desire to be a girl, which was most often confided to his mother, who was thereby extremely disturbed. Corresponding anxiety, loss of sexual desire for long periods, and extreme feelings of general incompetence were apparent in both of his parents. They had married young and were not only extremely infantilized late into adolescence by their own parents, but were still ambivalently dependent upon their own mothers during the greater part of our four years of therapeutic work with the family. For a long time these parents could not sleep together when the boy was home, because mother felt it necessary to sleep with him in order to calm him, by keeping her hand on his head, as he demanded, until he fell asleep.

Another instance involved an entirely mute boy who once cut his penis and frequently held his genitals in his hand when approaching nurses. His birth resulted from his mother's one extramarital affair, in which she had indulged because her husband's severe hypospadias and unsuccessful surgical repair precluded satisfactory intromission and coitus. A similar eleven-year-old, mute schizophrenic boy, perhaps the most extremely and most persistently isolated child in our experience, not only slept with his divorced mother, but also took showers with her.

We have learned during therapeutic work with mothers of other schizophrenic and neurotic children, especially girls, that the mothers felt extremely guilty about their own sexual responsiveness during bodily contact with their child. In each of these instances, the symptoms of the child included severe nocturnal terrors while sleeping with the mother or, in the cases of the hospitalized psychotic children, frequent open genital and anal masturbation, exposure of breasts, invitations addressed to nurses to perform cunnilingus upon them, and such acts as grabbing the nurses' breasts or legs, or lifting their skirts. In some of the neurotic girls, a primary symptom was obesity. In the instance of an early adolescent girl's episode of severe anorexia, alternating with marked obesity, the child told her therapist, towards the end of a thirty-month period of treatment, that her obese mother did not want her at home because her periodically alcoholic father tried to fondle his daughter's breasts.

The clinical data which I have outlined briefly in these vignettes and impressionistic statements do not, of course, form a sufficient basis for well-grounded theoretical formulations. They do, however, suggest the critical necessity of considering, in any effort to understand the genesis and maintenance of the child's disorder, the psychosexual actuality of both of his parents. It is important for me to know the experience with this actuality of any child who presents a clinical preoedipal or oedipal problem—whether this problem is overtly an impulsive character disorder, neurosis, or psychosis. In particular clinical instances, such facts of the parental, intraparental, and parent-child experiences concerning libidinous impulses may not require any important modification of therapeutic methods with the child himself. This is perhaps particularly true of the transference psychoneurotic disorders of childhood, where thorough, classical psychoanalysis of the child may be sufficiently efficacious.

THEORETICAL POSSIBILITIES

My impression from more than fifteen years of experience in psychiatric clinics for children is that in many of the severe, impulsive, and psychotic disorders of childhood, a concomitant psychotherapeutic effort which includes the parent, or better yet, both parents, may not only provide a more hopeful and sometimes a more effective therapy, but it may also provide the detailed clinical data upon which our theories of personality development and of etiology of the whole psychopathological spectrum may be made more precise and more specific.[2] Formulations based on such clinically obtained data concerning the earliest, pregenital vicissitudes of the child's libido, especially of its sadomasochistic transformations in the climate of parental regressions, may permit a clearer and mayhap simpler delineation of the factors, both inherited and experienced, which determine both the degree of ego-superego-id schisis, or malformation, and the degree of genitality, i.e., of intrapsychic integration, achieved by any human being. In particular, the role and nature of the incorporations of, introjections of, and identification with both parents, as actually experienced, and their phantastically revengeful, caricaturing, intrapsychic distortions, may be more obvious from the facts of a child's experience in his life situation. In sum, in our efforts to understand the most impulsive or the most bizarrely psychotic symptoms, we may then need less recourse to hypotheses—hitherto relatively unprovable in the individual case—of genetic constitutional factors. We might discover that the same factors which are sufficient to explain the clinical phenomenology of the transference neuroses are also sufficient (though quantitatively different in intensity and duration of action during the child's various developmental periods) to explain the impulsive and psychotic disorders.

If the child's genetic endowment is excluded from consideration for the moment, a tentative list of at least some of these more or less independently variable, experiential factors and their possible relations might read as follows:

1. The particular intensity and form of the neurosis which one or both parents bring, in their personality organization, from previous life experiences to the marriage or to the time of the child's birth.

2. The particular events in their marital history which constitute a stress or frustration to one or both parents, and which specifically, and quantitatively in combination, intensify the pre-existing and more or less latent parental neurosis. Among these I would include both those stresses determined wholly or in part by their neurotic tendencies, and those which occur independently of such tendencies, but which significantly affect them. Examples of the latter are: wars; general economic factors; somatic ill-

---

[2] In 1968, with nearly fifteen years' additional experience since this statement was made, I still find it essentially accurate.

nesses (their own or those of close relatives upon whom they are ambivalently dependent); the circumstances or time of birth of the child; and, the child's sex, intelligence, health, and general attractiveness.

3. The developmental phase or phases of the child during which he experiences the neurotic attitudes of his parents in response to those needs which are characteristic of his state of biological immaturity and helplessness. Because of the child's unsatisfactory experience during these phases, this factor determines the particular zonal fixations and the future libidinous regressions under later stress, the specificity of which is also here determined. The earlier the developmental phase, the deeper will be the later regression, other factors being equal.

4. The duration of operation of these factors which determine the intensity of the zonal libidinous fixations and the readiness of his later regressions. To put it in other terms: the longer the neurotogenic factors operate, the greater the fixation and the slighter the later stress or frustration which will precipitate regression.

5. The child's reaction to these factors is, of course, not only one of libidinous fixation, but also consists of the incorporations and introjections of, and identifications with, both parents' conscious and unconscious attitudes towards their own libidinous bodily tendencies which are reflected in their behavior—neurotic or integrated—toward each other and toward the child. These two factors, the libidinous fixations and the internalization of the parents' attitudes, determine which impulses of the child become egosyntonic and which are repressed. To the extent that these factors interfere with the child's satisfactory experience in any developmental phase, the internalized attitudes are revengefully (i.e., sadistically) caricatured and the libidinous impulses are masochistically distorted, i.e., the libidinous energy of both the id and the superego is fused with the rage and anxiety consequent to the repeated thwarting. It is here that Dr. Adelaide Johnson's phrase "superego lacunae" belongs. If the parental attitudes are not solidly integrated in their own personality organization—that is, if they are seriously ambivalent in their libidinous tendencies or manifest reaction-formations in regard to them—the child's identifications may combine in his own superego the lack of firmness and the corruptibility characteristic of both parents. The child's resulting disorder may then overtly appear to be more severe than that of either parent.

Necessarily, the other results of all these processes are: (1) ego malformation, of a degree directly proportional to these malintegrative processes, and (2) learning disability, which may

be specific or more generalized, as in mute, very isolated schizophrenic children or in the impulsive character disorders. As we
know in both of these disorders, later experience, even with persons other than the parents, is integrated only slightly, if at all.
The typically poor prognosis for response to the usual form of
analytic therapy is, I think, another indication of the severity of the
pathology.

6. It is perhaps hardly necessary to add that this neurotic
development of the child's personality has a further potentiating,
neurotogenic effect upon the parents' neuroses. It is the presence
of these vicious circles established between the parents and between them and their child which, to me, often constitutes the
indication for simultaneous therapeutic work with mother, father,
and child.

Finally, it seems to me that the time in the family history when
these factors occur and their particular combination determine
not only which child develops the pathology—if only one of several
in a family is primarily affected—but also what form his disorder
will take.

REFERENCES

1. BERLIN, I. N., BOATMAN, M. J., SHEIMO, S. L., & SZUREK,
S. A. Adolescent alternation of anorexia and obesity, Am. J. Ortho-
psychiat., 21:387-419, 1951. Reprinted in S. A. Szurek & I. N.
Berlin (Eds.), Psychosomatic disorders and mental retardation in
children. Vol. 3, the Langley Porter Child Psychiatry Series. Palo
Alto, Calif.: Science and Behavior Books, 1967.

2. FABIAN, A. A., & HOLDEN, M. A. Treatment of childhood
schizophrenia in a child guidance clinic, Am. J. Orthopsychiat.,
21:571-581, 1951.

3. GIFFIN, M. E., JOHNSON, A. M., & LITLIN, E. M. Parental
seduction as related to acting out in young and adolescent children.
Paper read at the American Psychoanalytic Association, New York,
December, 1953.

4. JOHNSON, A. M. Sanctions for superego lacunae of adolescents. In K. R. Eissler (Ed.), Searchlights on delinquency. New
York: International Universities Press, 1949.

5. JOHNSON, A. M., FALSTEIN, E. I., SZUREK, S. A., &
SVENDSEN, M. School phobia. Am. J. Orthopsychiat., 11:702-711,
1941. Reprinted in I. N. Berlin & S. A. Szurek (Eds.), Learning
and its disorders. Vol. 1, the Langley Porter Child Psychiatry
Series. Palo Alto, Calif.: Science and Behavior Books, 1965.

6. JOHNSON, A. M., & SZUREK, S. A. The genesis of antisocial acting out in children and adults. Psychoanal. Quart., 21:323-343, 1952. Reprinted in I. N. Berlin & S. A. Szurek (Eds.), Learning and its disorders. Vol. 1, the Langley Porter Child Psychiatry Series. Palo Alto, Calif.: Science and Behavior Books, 1965.

7. PUTNAM, M., et al. Case study of an atypical two-and-a-half-year-old. Am. J. Orthopsychiat., 18:1-30, 1948

8. RANK, B. Adaption of the psychoanalytic technique for the treatment of young children with atypical development. Am. J. Orthopsychiat., 19:130-139, 1949.

9. SPERLING, M. Analysis of case of recurrent ulcer of the leg. Psychoanal. Study of the Child. New York: International Universities Press, 1949.

10. SPERLING, M. Problems in analysis of children with psychosomatic disorders. Quart. J. Child Behavior, 1:12-17, 1949.

11. SPERLING, M. Neurotic sleep disturbances in children. Nerv. Child, 8:28-46, 1949.

12. SPERLING, M. The role of the mother in psychosomatic disorders in children. Psychosom. Med., 11:377-385, 1949.

13. SPERLING, M. Mucuous colitis associated with phobias. Psychoanal. Quart., 19:318-326, 1950.

14. SPERLING, M. The neurotic child and its mother: A psychoanalytic study, Am. J. Orthopsychiat., 21:351-364, 1951.

15. SZUREK, S. A. Notes on the genesis of psychopathic personality trends, Psychiatry, 5:1-6, 1942. (See page 3 of this volume.)

16. SZUREK, S. A. An attitude towards (child) psychiatry. Quart. J. Child Behavior, 1:22-54, 178-213, 375-399, 401-423, 1949. Reprinted in S. A. Szurek & I. N. Berlin (Eds.), Training in Work with Children. Vol. 2, the Langley Porter Child Psychiatry Series. Palo Alto, Calif.: Science and Behavior Books, 1967.

17. SZUREK, S. A. Some impressions from clinical experience with delinquents. In K. R. Eissler (Ed.), Searchlights on Delinquency. New York: International Universities Press, 1949. (See page 72 of this volume.)

18. SZUREK, S. A. Remarks on training for psychotherapy, Am. J. Orthopsychiat., 19:36-51, 1949. Reprinted in S. A. Szurek & I. N. Berlin (Eds.), Training in Therapeutic Work with Children. Vol. 2, the Langley Porter Child Psychiatry Series. Palo Alto, Calif.: Science and Behavior Books, 1967.

19. SZUREK, S. A. The family and the staff in hospital psychiatric therapy of children. Am. J. Orthopsychiat., 21:597-611, 1951.

20. SZUREK, S. A. "Critique" in chapter on Langley Porter Clinic Children's Inpatient Service. In J. H. Reid & H. R. Hagen, (Eds.), Residential Treatment of Emotionally Disturbed Children, New York: Child Welfare League of America, 1952.

21. SZUREK, S. A. Some lessons from efforts at psychotherapy with parents, Am. J. Psychiat., 109:296-302, 1952. Reprinted in S. A. Szurek & I. N. Berlin (Eds.), Training in Therapeutic Work with Children. Vol. 2, the Langley Porter Child Psychiatry Series. Palo Alto, Calif.: Science and Behavior Books, 1967.

22. SZUREK, S. A., JOHNSON, A. M., & FALSTEIN, E. I. Collaborative psychiatric therapy of parent-child problems. Am. J. Orthopsychiat., 12:511-516, 1942. Reprinted in S. A. Szurek & I. N. Berlin (Eds.), Training in Therapeutic Work with Children. Vol. 2, the Langley Porter Child Psychiatry Series. Palo Alto, Calif.: Science and Behavior Books, 1967.

SECTION TWO

THE QUESTION OF AUTHORITY AND CONTROLS

INTRODUCTION

A very obvious problem with respect to antisocial behavior in children is the problem of authority as exercised by parents toward them. The internalization of this experience in which such authority is exercised is then manifested as an inner control, self-direction, and capacity for discriminations and choice in the child's behavior.

The vicissitudes in the exercise and experience of authority in a variety of life situations and its importance in therapeutic work are examined in the following two chapters.

EMOTIONAL FACTORS IN THE USE OF AUTHORITY*

S. A. Szurek

There is perhaps no more troublesome problem than that of authority, not only in interpersonal situations where two or more persons have relations with one other, but also in those situations where larger groups of people—especially nations—interact. It is not necessary here to say much to substantiate this statement. Such words and phrases as "civil rights," "dictatorship," "democracy," "totalitarianism," "police state," "the sovereignty of a nation," "freedom"—to name only a few—will recall to your mind the manifold problems of authority which acutely beset us now in the world, and which probably beset every generation in human history.

Some might object that such problems are far removed from the purpose of this book. These are political problems, one might say, or problems in philosophy, or in political science, or in law; or at best they are the phenomena of human historical processes. Certainly, such an objector could maintain, the problem of authority has only a tangential relation to science, to medicine, or to one of its specialties, psychiatry. Nevertheless, if we can succeed in convincing you that psychiatry has something to do with the problems of people living together, with their influence upon one another, even with their effect upon one another's health and bodily functions, then it will be quite obvious that no medical man can be unconcerned about the problem of authority. Whether the doctor is clearly aware of the problem or not, he is constantly involved in its implications. This is true simply because he himself is vested with a certain authority. He is vested with this authority not only by virtue of his medical license and degree, but also by virtue of the feelings of his patients toward him. And in public health work special, legally established responsibilities of the medical officer invest him with an authority in certain situations which differs in

*Reprinted with permission from Public Health Is People, published by The Commonwealth Fund, New York, 1950, pp. 206-225.

its nature and problems from those of the physician in private practice. How he exercises this authority is of tremendous importance for the effectiveness of his work and for his own satisfaction in it.

I shall probably never forget a bit of autobiography one of my teachers in medical school shared with us. He said it took him ten years in private practice to unlearn what he had acquired in his work with charity patients during his internship in a county hospital. During those first ten years of practice, he examined conscientiously, studied thoroughly, and prescribed sometimes minutely for his patients. If a patient returned some months later no better for his ministrations and occasionally even worse off, and if he learned that the patient had taken one of his prescriptions but failed even to have another prescription filled, he became angry and offended. He ordered the patient to leave and seek another physician's help. Gradually it dawned on him that the motto of the salesman, "The customer is always right," was equally applicable to the practice of medicine. If the patient had asked, received, and paid for a doctor's advice, he really had the right to do with it what he wished—which, of course, included the right to disregard it. After he had learned the lesson it took him a decade of medical practice to acquire, my teacher thereafter, with regretful but more sympathetic patience, tried to unravel the again-tangled threads of his patient's illness.

This story illustrates very dramatically for me many of the frequent problems with regard to authority involved in the physician-patient relationship. It suggests some sources of our later difficulties with effective medical practice. It describes a too frequent attitude which complicates work with patients and generally diminishes therapeutic influence. An older colleague of mine, himself a psychiatrist, once humorously described a psychiatrist as a doctor who could rarely, if ever, be insulted. The wisecrack has an important half-truth in it.

Another illustration of the same kind of difficulty—a personal experience from my own early efforts at psychotherapy—comes to mind. It was in the days when I hoped that I had learned enough of psychotherapy from reading and lectures to be able to seem useful, and certainly informed, to patients. One patient in particular continued to come to see me for a much longer time than the circumstances seemed to warrant. I listened for many sessions with a studied, and to me quite frequently strained, silence until an explanation of his behavior—a "mechanism," as we were then prone to call it—dawned on me. With insufficiently restrained enthusiasm, if not glee, I pronounced an interpretation to the patient. He listened politely and again effectively reduced me to strained silence by the brief reply, "So what!" Although I was not clear about it then, I later realized that my patient and I were struggling about authority. The interpretation meant nothing to him subjectively, and yet I expected him to accept it wholeheartedly on my say-so.

Many years later, after I had undergone considerable discipline during training for psychoanalytic therapy, a patient of Central European origin listened with obvious uneasiness to the note of annoyance and impatience in my voice as I commented on what he was saying for the twentieth-or-more time. He interposed with anxious amazement that I sounded very angry. After I promptly acknowledged that I was annoyed and told him why, he said with evident relief, but persistent astonishment, that he had the impression from previous European experience that "Analytikers" did not have, much less did they display, any feelings toward their patients. This patient had had problems of authority and was still struggling vainly with them, but at this time I felt much less uneasy about mine.

I would like to add one more illustrative anecdote. This was a personal experience during my first month as an intern, when a ward patient gave me my first, startlingly unexpected experience and minor success in psychotherapy. After a gynecological laparotomy this woman was placed in a quiet room. Her own surgery was uncomplicated, and her post-operative course was expected to be smooth. It was my duty as junior intern to make daily urinalyses until the post-operative acidosis disappeared. On a busy service it became a bit troublesome, as well as a matter of considerable concern, when the acetone and diacetic acid tests remained four-plus on the third and fourth days. I investigated and learned from the nurses that the patient was afraid to drink and eat because her roommate, who had eviscerated following her first intake of fluids by mouth about a week before, lay distended in the other bed still in acute discomfort with a stomach tube protruding from her lips. I tried more or less gently to reassure the first patient that nothing like that threatened her, that her wound was healing well, that her general condition was excellent and would improve if only she would begin to take fluids. On the fifth and sixth days the acidosis was practically undiminished; the patient continued to be uneasy about fluid intake. The pressure of my work increased, as did my concern for the patient. I spoke again to the patient, this time with more annoyance than I wished, telling her I saw no need for her attitude and behavior, that there were reasons for her roommate's condition other than the intake of fluids post-operatively. By the following day the acidosis had completely disappeared.

For my part, I was a bit ashamed of my assumption of a paternal tone toward a woman a decade or more my senior. I avoided her somewhat for my remaining few days on the service and on the last day was quite uneasy about saying good-bye to her, as I did to all the other patients on the ward. However, in spite of my discomfort, I did say good-bye and tried to turn away quickly. I was amazed to find that one of my hands was suddenly grasped by both of hers and kissed. With tears in her eyes and with quite obviously genuine gratitude, the woman thanked me and said that I had done more for her than anyone else in the hospital! This was my first clinical lesson in the therapeutic power of authority. Apparently the patient was more impressed with my interest and concern for her welfare than resentful of the impatience of which I had been so ashamed.

What are some of the elements common to all these situations? Is there more than one kind of authority? Are all situations involving authority equally unpleasant and likely to cause difficulty for both the person in authority and the subordinate? Are these difficulties inevitable? Or are there tendencies on both sides which may spell the difference between a mutually happy and effective relation and one which is full of trouble and discomfort?

TYPES OF AUTHORITY

Merely to ask these questions is to suggest some of the answers. We know that despite the frequency of trouble in the relations between a superior and a subordinate there are instances in which all kinds of authority are effectively exercised with willing and happy cooperation on the part of subordinates. Now and then we also see some peculiar relationships. We ask ourselves then how a person can take such attitudes from the so-and-so. Or we wonder how someone can be so mean. Yet both parties may not only appear content, but each may actually defend or even extol the situation or the other person. It is easy for most of us to understand why the dominant one might be satisfied in such peculiar relationships. It is more difficult for us to comprehend what the apparent underdog, who seems happy, gets out of it, or how he got that way.

Suggestions have been made and explanations given regarding these same problems in other contexts, so that some of what I say now will be repetitious. But perhaps this repetition may not be altogether useless.

It is possible—according to Erich Fromm(1)—to distinguish two general types of interpersonal situations in which authority plays a role, though only rarely do we meet either type in its pure form, especially in this country with its traditions and ethics. These two types are polar opposites, and may represent the limits along a scale of variation never actually reached, like the asymptotes of a hyperbola. In other words, we may be making a distinction between the absolute good and the absolute bad, the angel and the devil, and hence may not be describing reality as it actually occurs in interpersonal integrations. Nevertheless, I have found the conceptions of these two types of authority situations to be useful in my thinking and practice, provided I also remember to define how much of each type is present in any actual instance.

These two types of authority-subordinate relationships can be distinguished by mode of operation, basic purpose, and predominant or usual outcome.

In one type of relationship—which might be called authoritarian—coercive power, whatever its nature, is exercised by the dominant person primarily for his own rather than the subordinate's immediate gain. The power is exercised to the end that the status quo of the relation be continued forever, or for as long as possible. In simpler terms it is an enslavement, an effort by the dominant person to maintain control of the slave's services, deference, admiration, or whatever is demanded. Only such care is given, only such concessions or attention to the inferior person's welfare and needs are made, as will enhance or assure the continuation of the benefits and profit to the more dominant person. Certainly there is neither concern nor interest in developing the inferior's potential abilities or strength, for this might endanger the relationship or lead to freedom for the inferior. On the contrary, there is positive hostility and fear of such a possibility, often on the part of both persons. What is little realized is that personal stultification is inevitable for both persons. As one writer puts it, every dictator is slavish and every slave dictatorial. There are other describable results of this type of relationship, such as ruthless cruelty, mutual suspicions, hostilities, rebelliousness, retaliatory anxieties and chronic tensions which produce great anxiety about prestige, brittle rigidity of attitudes, and a narrow pessimistic outlook.

In the opposite type of authority-subordinate relation—which might be called democratic or more legitimately authoritative—the converse is observed in all these characteristics. Coercion is absent: the authority derives from superior competence and skill. As in the best teacher-student or ideal parent-child relations, the purpose of both persons in the situation is to promote and foster the subordinate's acquisition of the competence and skill of the authority. Their common effort is to grow more alike in respect to the power which the competence brings and eventually to achieve equality and genuine freedom of each other. Admiration and deep respect is mutual. Confidence, optimism, and benign expansive-

ness of outlook, readiness for experimentation and risk, and a
tolerance for thwarting, frustrating obstacles as well as a capacity
for more enthusiastically productive work are characteristic
qualities generated in such relations. Rather than envy, the good
teacher or ideal parent manifests genuine delight if the student or
child approaches or even begins to surpass his own competence.
Sympathy without any trace of contemptuous pity and mutually affectionate warmth without anxious oversolicitude permeate the relationship. Flexibility of attitudes, coupled with firm consistency, is
gradually transmitted from the authority to the subordinate.

There are many other contrasts between these two extremes of
authority relations. What has been called spiritual anthropophagia
of authoritarian type is replaced by anthropophilia of the democratic or authoritative type. This is, of course, a polysyllabic way
of saying that destructive, emotional swallowing of man by man is
supplanted by genuine love of man.

This distinction requires us to make some very necessary dis-
tinctions between varieties of "love." Many relationships essentially of the dictator-slave variety are called "love" even—perhaps
especially—by the participants. When sexual activities occur in
these situations, one may be certain that they will belong to the
sado-masochistic category, regardless of what bodily zones or
orifices are stimulated and regardless of the sex of both persons.
The fact that jealousy and exclusive possessiveness (as well as
depressions, panics, or impulses to murder or suicide on threatened separations) are so widely accepted as natural concomitants
of "love" is no justification to perpetuate the unconscious self-
deception that mutual enslavement has anything in common with a
mature, genuine love. Mature love, it has been said, has no need
to be blind. When one loves maturely, one loves the other person
in spite of the qualities one dislikes in him.

THE MATURE AUTHORITY FIGURE

Emotional maturity capable of such love is an expression of a
self-love which is clear-eyed and tolerant of the limitations within
oneself; at the same time it is contentedly and securely proud of
one's assets. Such self-love cannot be mistaken for the deeply
anxious concern about the self which must disguise its self-
destructive sense of terrible inferiority and weakness either with
a brittle and aloof conceit (and an exaggerated appearance of supe-
riority) or with an ingratiatingly submissive self-abnegation and an
assumed false modesty. It is probably this very great feeling of
inferiority and weakness, however hidden from others or unconscious to the self, which is the source of, and chief motivational

energy behind, the compensatory drive for power over others which leads to the dictatorial, enslaving types of relationships. A genuine and solid self-love cannot be depleted by love of another. On the contrary it is enhanced, and sacrifices or services to the other flow from relatively inexhaustible reserves of strength and plenty. Such self-respect neither countenances domination nor requires submission from another. In other words, there is neither masochism nor sadism, neither slavishness nor tyranny. By its nature it fosters the growth of the potentialities of the other and revels in the give and take between equals. By its very nature and needs it cannot behave otherwise. Hence, without strain or effort on the part of such a person, all others who come in contact with such qualities of personality are attracted and so affected as to make even some tiny steps toward maturity and freedom themselves.

Maturity is not at all immune to a tragic sense of life. It is not, for instance, immune to genuine grief and mourning for the loss of a beloved person through death. It is not, however, subject to the likelihood of the severe depressions or agitatedly depressive reactions of the authoritarian-dependent character in the event of the death of, or temporary separation from, the person with whom it is enmeshed. In these depressive reactions, of course, exaggerated fears about one's future, fears of loneliness, and guilt about one's hostilities toward the other person are prominent. In both types of character there is an identification with the other and an incorporation of the other into one's own ego or self. But the treatment of this incorporated object and, in turn, the effect of the incorporated object upon the self are quite opposite, and the resultant feelings differ markedly. Instead of panic, or anxiety, or the repression and splitting off of these emotions, there is ready expression of sadness, grief, and longing. Instead of the schizoid absence of feeling in consciousness, resulting from a repression of panic and anxiety, with its attendant sense of impoverishment of the self and unbearable loneliness, helplessness, and futility, there is a fullness of feeling, however painful, and with its full expression there comes a calm enrichment within the self with positively toned memories of the other.

Thus, in the case of the mature person, there is no panicky sense of loss or abandonment when the other is temporarily absent. He still has contact with the other through pleasant memories and through continuing affectionate feelings, despite great geographical separation and infrequent communication. In other words the mature person has a feeling of wholeness and no sense of diminution of his power or strength. With the immature person, however, the opposite is the case. There is a kind of fragmentation of the self with an inevitable increase in the inability to deal with the reality of his own actual assets and potentialities, and with the reality of the friendliness of other persons remaining about him.

The mature person has no Pollyanna quality in his recovering optimism. He has, instead, a capacity for realistic discrimination of the possibilities in the actual situation after his loss. The bereaved, genuinely loving person carries on. The slavish-dictatorial person tends to collapse, to reduce his activities in the real world of remaining persons. At least his hedonism or enjoyment is reduced. He senses within himself a futility and gloom. An uncanny world of terrors and unnamed threats frequently obscures the actual world of other persons and the possibilities for personal satisfaction. One retains or rapidly regains possession of himself; the other tends to lose his grip on himself, go to pieces, feel a progressive sense of unreality; sometimes he progresses to a state of depersonalization. In such circumstances the mature person actually requires solitude; but even at other times he serenely enjoys his own companionship. The immature, the authoritarian person, on the other hand, carries within him a deep sense of estrangement from himself—the result, in psychoanalytic terms, of the hateful tension between the superego and the ego—such a sense of constant loneliness and bereavement that solitude is intolerable.

Another difference between these extremely opposite personalities is that the genuinely friendly, mature person, unlike the other, has no need for exclusiveness in his affectionate ties with people. Feeling a good deal of warmth and tenderness for several persons in no way diminishes the intensity of his feeling for a few intimate friends or for the especially beloved person of the opposite sex. The immature personality, however, compulsively attaches himself to one other person with such tremendous all-consuming force that relations with others are rarely as intense and are generally incompatible with it. Automatically and rather helplessly he puts all his eggs in one basket, hence any slight threat to this basket tends to precipitate feelings of impending cosmic disaster.

One could go on and on through the whole gamut of variations in human psychopathology to show that the personality traits of the participants—that is, the emotional factors in the relationship—determine the quality of any authority exercised. Perhaps, however, I have indicated enough of the background to bring into focus the problems suggested by the title of this chapter.

CONFLICT IN AUTHORITY RELATIONSHIPS

Conflict between persons generally occurs whenever an egocentric impulse of one person meets opposition to its gratification from another person in authority. The impulse may be for some necessary bodily satisfaction or for some more psychological (emotional) need for security, prestige, affection, approval, or the like. The opposition to gratification may be motivated by various factors, perhaps most often by an inability to supply the need; anxiety about being deprived or hurt by the demand; or ideally, as in the case of a parent in regard to a child's impulse, by genuine interest in the person's immediate safety or future welfare. This latter problem—the concern of the person in authority for the immediate and future welfare of the subordinate—is, of course, part of a much wider problem: the satisfactory adjustment of the quite individual needs of each person and his welfare to the needs and welfare of the group of which he is a part. In guiding individual persons toward ways of gratifying their egocentric impulses that will be either less destructive to, or more in consonance with, the welfare of the entire group, one has something of the parent's problem of inculcating durable personality traits in the child that will fit him to live happily and responsibly within his culture.

In any case, whenever such opposition to egocentric impulses is encountered and for whatever reasons, anger is generally the inevitable and biologically adequate reaction. Under such circumstances a healthy organism, human or not, reacts not only with rage but also with efforts to circumvent or remove the obstacles to its satisfactions. If this is impossible, there is a revengeful attack upon the opposing organism. Whether this rage or attack is direct or indirect, frank or disguised, and whether or not it is persistent depends, of course, on many factors, not the least of which is the relative strength and power of the two persons involved. Another factor of great importance to the eventual resolution of such a conflict is the firmness of the person in authority. This firmness is very frequently a crucial factor in the manner in which the conflict is solved. It frequently determines whether the subordinate learns how to get satisfactions in ways which are nondestructive to himself and others, or whether he remains rebelliously set in seeking his own satisfactions quite egocentrically, disregarding the welfare of others. In the latter case he may also remain distrustful of all authority, with a suspicious, hostile readiness to react defensively and often self-destructively to any suggestions from others. He then remains unintegrated with the group, in effect isolated from it, perhaps maintaining an exaggerated self-assertiveness which further estranges him from others and which estranges others still further from him.

FIRMNESS IN THE AUTHORITY FIGURE

For these reasons the quality of firmness in the authoritative person is very important and requires more detailed examination.

In the first place, firmness needs to be distinguished from dictatorial or sadistic suppression, deprivation, or complete denial of any gratification to the subordinate. In brief, the authority does not assert himself in the conflict situation merely for the sake of an egocentric satisfaction of his own power and prestige. His primary purpose is not to deny all satisfaction to the subordinate's impulse, but to guide him in obtaining satisfaction in ways which are nondestructive to the interests of others or to his own other self-interests. His purpose is to indicate ways which will ultimately gain for the subordinate deeper satisfaction, since they will tend to integrate him with the social group whose approval enhances his self-esteem. Such firmness on the part of the authority, then, is possible when, and only when, the authoritative person's conscience is clear as to his motives in regard to the welfare of the subordinate. If he has no need to deprive the subordinate, if he has no egocentric (compensatory) power drives or exaggerated prestige needs of his own, if he has no wish to enslave the other or hurt him revengefully, he will be free of retaliatory anxieties. He can then remain calmly and quietly firm in opposition, not to the impulse of the subordinate, but to the manner or circumstances of its satisfaction.

There are other describable and essential elements which contribute to the quality of firmness on the part of an authority. Perhaps the chief one of these is that the authoritative person himself is integrated, is wholehearted in his own attitude with regard to the impulse active in the subordinate. In other words, it appears to me necessary that the authority himself has actually learned ways of gratifying such an impulse in accordance with his self-esteem and the mores and ethics of the social group. This again presupposes that one might call emotional maturity, a mastery of exactly similar impulses within himself. By mastery of impulses I do not imply simply a constantly uncertain, although sometimes fanatically rigid, self-restraint, a compensatory reaction formation. Such compensatory attitudes, opposite in direction to the given impulse, generally signify that the conflict is active and persistent. In situations affording temptation or the possibility of gratification, the balance of forces within the self remains precarious. Under these circumstances of unresolved conflict—even though the conflict is largely or wholly unconscious—within the personality of the authoritative person, the pressure or the demand of the impulse of the subordinate often increases the conflict. The authority is usually uneasy and tends to vacillate within himself about prohibiting another from doing what he is either tempted or actually permits himself to do.

Such anxiety tends to cloud the issue with the subordinate and often leads the authority to irrational behavior in order to deal with his own anxiety: he is either doubtful and hesitant, or defensively

authoritarian and suppressive. Neither type of reaction can be
called firmness. If the authority vacillates, the tendency of the
subordinate is to gratify his impulse even though surreptitiously.
If the authority is defensively suppressive and dictatorial, defiant
self-assertiveness is likely to be aroused in the subordinate.
Whether the subordinate responds to either attitude in these ways
or in some other manner depends, of course, on his character, on
his previous experience with authority and the patterns of behavior
he has previously acquired in these experiences, and on other possibilities in the actual current situation. In any case, the subordinate is likely to experience anxiety in reaction to the anxiety of the
authority. Anxiety in a serious degree in any person tends to fog
his perception of the realities of the situation and of his own self-
interest.

Another element in the quality of firmness is patience. The person who has matured emotionally, who has genuinely resolved the
conflicts of his earlier life, not only is convinced through his own
experience that it is quite often possible to gratify one's selfish
impulses nondestructively, but is also convinced through such personal experience that it takes time to achieve such solutions. He
has learned among other things that emergencies are relatively
rare in peacetime, that most problems are capable of solution, that
even though he may not see how to meet a threat to his satisfactions at a given moment, a solution may appear later. He has
learned that no miracles are necessary in such instances but that a
"miraculous" clarification of the situation and of his own feelings
can occur if only he first grants himself time to see how he feels
about the dilemma and to examine more closely what real possibilities exist. He realizes that his own rage at the threatened
thwarting need not be destructive to anyone, since he has learned
well that he can control the form of its expression. He has learned
finally that his whole happiness never depends upon the loss of any
one satisfaction and that he can survive it. To him the whole world
of other persons rarely appears as totally hostile, unjust, or op-
pressive. At the same time, having lived through such anxieties,
impatience, greediness, and subjective cosmic calamities in his
own progress toward maturing, he appreciates sympathetically
what the subordinate is experiencing. This sympathetic appreciation permits him to wait patiently, but none the less firmly, for the
subordinate to make alternative choices of action. His quiet confidence, reflecting his own achievement, is then a positive, constructive aid to the subordinate, who psychologically and often unconsciously imbibes of it.

I have been discussing the problems and difficulties of the person in authority. This is in many respects the converse of the

"what is wrong with the patient" type of discussion, which is more usual in discourses on psychopathology. This discussion does not mean that I feel that all the difficulty in authority-subordinate relationships resides on one side of such relationships, nor that if the person in authority were only more thoroughly integrated emotionally and more mature, all problems would end. The role of the patient or subordinate in these relationship difficulties is considerable; it has been implied and touched upon here and in other chapters. The entire range of immature tendencies—the regressive attitudes of helplessness; the demand for protection, for care, for relief from all responsibilities; the slavish ingratiation used to obtain gratification; and many other attitudes—are here involved. But I have been interested in making two points: first, that immaturity does not by itself progress to maturity, but requires mature help, guidance, and firmness from another; and second, that the difficulties between two people rarely stem from the immaturities of only one of them.

AUTHORITY IN THE THERAPEUTIC RELATIONSHIP

This latter point brings me to the final topic of this chapter. I have already suggested that the critically important factor is how much immaturity remains and how much maturity has been achieved by any one of us at a given period of his life. The dynamic balance between these two constitutes our total self-organization or personality. Whether we are aware of our immature tendencies or not, whether we are conscious either of the regressive trends or of our defenses against them makes little difference. If they constitute an important fraction of our total attitudes toward ourselves, they will be evident in certain interpersonal situations. They will be stirred up or intensified to disturb us and the other person. Our tendencies to irrational behavior, our anxieties and underlying conflicts are particularly apt to be aroused in situations involving authority and in love relationships. In the case of those relations where authority is involved, our conflicts may be equally heightened in the position of either authority or subordinate.

From this point of view it is obvious that periods of neurotic illness and disorder may be precipitated in our patients, and in ourselves, by situations involving persons in authority, persons with whom the patient is currently "in love," or both types of persons. It is then that people become our patients whether we are psychiatrists or not.

This is not the place to review in any detail what the therapy consists of, whether it be in a psychiatrist's office or in the office of the nonpsychiatric medical practitioner. However, one may mention a few of the steps which one hopes will occur. The first phase of such interaction is the establishment of a working rapport—the transference, a relationship between patient and doctor with therapeutic potentialities. This has many rather technical problems. One is the time such a transference may require, and another is the basic attitude of the doctor, leaving out of consideration the character of the patient. Both of these are variable from patient to patient and from physician to physician. That is, the time required generally varies inversely with the skill, experience, and basic attitude of the doctor. The greater his skill, experience, and maturity, the shorter the time required (other things being equal, such as the frequency of visits, age, and character problem of the patients).

There follows, with no sharp line of demarcation from the first phase, the phase of "working through." This in reality is a repetition of the inevitable struggles of the patient both to reestablish and to maintain a relationship characteristic of his degree of immaturity, and to resolve the conflict between the immature and mature portions of his total self. The result or outcome of this phase varies, of course, and depends on many factors. Certainly, even in the most intensive efforts at psychotherapy, namely, in psychoanalytic treatment, no perfectionistic goals are attainable or necessary. Although in psychoanalytic therapy the hope is that the character of the patient, the total self or personality, may undergo a rather basic reorganization, a great deal has been accomplished if at least some firm steps are taken in this direction. If only a few limitations to growth are removed or even just loosened, much has been achieved. The only factor I wish to emphasize again is the attitude, the actual maturity, the competence of the doctor. If his authority is based on such competence and if it is infused with at least a measure of the parental desire to help and to allow the patient to grow, then movement toward the common goal of doctor and patient may occur.

We can, in conclusion, briefly examine the specific problem of the utilization of authority in the situation of an executive or director and his staff. Although some of the same processes may occur, although some of the same dynamics may be present in this situation as in the therapeutic relationship, there are a few obvious differences. For one thing, the complexity in executive-staff relations is obviously greater. One enters the sphere of larger social integrations, of group psychology, and of leadership. The interrelations and problems between the subordinates, either as equals or between levels of a hierarchy of authority, are present. Mutual envies and competitions, as well as sibling-like collaboration, are present. In this collaboration there occur interidentifications, which in effect are identification with the leader for the purpose of the organization's work. Nevertheless, interidentifications for mutual support in rebellion against the leader may at times be predominant or co-exist with the whole collaborative attitude. Problems of delegation of responsibility and authority always exist. The degree of freedom granted the subordinate and the encouragement of his independent decisions within the limits of the delegated authority are obviously important.

The problem frequently arises of how to avoid making punitive changes in general policy that affect all members of the staff when only one member fails to act responsibly. Questions of group morale occur. These are frequently, if not generally, questions of the nature of the leadership and the type of authority exercised by the director. His attention to reward by approval, appreciation, or promotion is as important as his promptness of censure and disapproval. Perhaps of even greater importance is the leader's actual competence in all phases of the organization's work and his willingness to risk being wrong. The latter quality frequently relieves much anxiety in the subordinates about their inadequacies, inexperience, and incompetence. It may release whatever growth potential exists in them.

Finally, the leader's readiness to accept specific competences of a subordinate which may be superior to his own is of great importance. For the leader to accept a subordinate who has grown and matured in skill as an equal and as a colleague and for the leader always deeply and spontaneously to respect the subordinate's personality remain the most effective incentives for each individual subordinate and provide the integrating power for the entire staff as a unit. Authority so exercised is likely to meet a minimum of interference from complicating or obstructing emotional factors.

REFERENCES

1. Fromm, E. Escape from freedom. New York: Rinehart, 1941.

CONTROLS: THEIR CONTRIBUTION
TO CORRECTIVE LEARNING*

Samuel Susselman

Concepts of authority are implicit in the work and philosophy of
psychiatric clinics and other community agencies. At critical
times, however, difficulties arise in the use of controls. This is
especially true of the law enforcer and the correctional worker,
who, while coping with the most urgent of all community problems,
sometimes question whether their use of controls is therapeutic.

A unique opportunity to study the interpersonal ramifications in
the use of authority under pressure occurs in the course of psychotherapy in the playroom with children whose behavior can reach
destructive proportions. Children, unlike adults in treatment, are
expected and encouraged to express themselves through physical
activity in the form of play. As a result, therapists, like correctional workers, often are confronted with the imperative need to
make quick decisions and to act promptly and precisely when behavior becomes destructive. Otherwise they risk personal harm,
damage to property, or injury to self-esteem with resultant dete-
rioration in the therapeutic work. The use of physical restraint in
these critical instances has taught us that the exercise of control
primarily to protect ourselves is compatible with helping the individual who will not or cannot control his destructive behavior. Let
us start this presentation by the following fragment of an experience in the playroom:

My patient turned to the finger paints, and I hoped he would
limit himself to one or two of the six colors. He dipped the wooden
tongue blade into the jar of red paint and transferred a huge glob of
expendable paint to a clean sheet of expendable paper. Things
seemed to be going smoothly as I helped him tap all the paint off
the stick. He then turned eagerly to the jar of yellow paint, but to
avoid contamination with the red, I asked him to wait until I could
wash off the tongue blade.

---

*Unpublished, 1957.

(Only the day before I had observed one of my colleagues and a patient in the playroom: all six jars of paint were open and each contained a tongue blade. I liked this method but I hesitated to adopt it because I might thus encourage my patient to follow his usual custom of taking paint from all the jars. Consequently I persisted with the one tongue blade, pausing to clean it each time and hoping he would not run the gamut of colors. In a dim way I was aware that when he made a move towards the finger paints something unpleasant happened to me. I do not like a mess in the first place and six blades meant six times the mess. Besides, my French cuffs, smudged with paint once before, were too long and again in danger. In addition, I wore no protective covering for my freshly cleaned suit, since the therapist who had used the playroom the preceding hour had left the solitary smock so soaking wet that I could not wear it. I was angry with him not only because the smock was unusable but because this had happened before. I was also angry with myself because I had intended to mention it to him but had forgotten to do so. Furthermore, I had meant to provide myself with a smock but had forgotten to do that, too. I had once inquired about securing clean gowns and was told that they were not part of playroom equipment: finger paint stained them beyond washability, and it was only through the kindness of the housekeeper that we had any gowns at all. I was advised not to raise the subject with her for I might spoil a good thing. I had considered buying my own smock but could not find time to shop for it. The truth was that I was reluctant to pay for it myself. Why did the clinic not buy one for me, anyhow! Even if I owned one I had no good place to hide it in the crowded office I shared with several others. Where would it be safe from another therapist in search of a clean smock? How would I get it laundered, and what would I wear while it was being washed? Should I buy two smocks? After all this speculation I had deferred the whole matter and there I was in the playroom again with no protection for my clothes.)

On opening the jar of yellow paint we found that it was already contaminated by the blue. How could I insist that my patient be meticulously careful? Suddenly I felt how picayune I must have seemed to him. Very apologetically, I explained why I had voiced restrictions, but I did not sound very convincing.

Encouraging a child to play as a means of his expressing himself and of our helping him to work out problems was not a simple matter for me that day. Almost predictably, his play became more and more hectic. Finger paint splattered the counter, the walls, the floor, and me. The child too was a mess. (It may not surprise you that while all this was happening, I was not clearly aware of all the details I have just recounted. I was too busy with my own preoccupations and with the child to attend to them. Only later was I able to piece things together for a retrospective learning experience.)

Since that episode I come to the playroom appropriately dressed for the occasion. On those days when it is not convenient to wear old clothes or when a gown is not available, I can say quite easily to my patient that he will have to be especially careful because I do not want to be smeared with paint. His response has been gratifying. He uses the finger paints enjoyably and within bounds. Constant alertness is still necessary to deal with early signs of rebellious behavior, but now a restraining word is usually sufficient where formerly a restraining hand was of no avail. It has been a mutual learning experience.

From such incidents it becomes clear that the decision of when and how to use controls depends on many variables. How the therapist acts (or does not act) is a function of his own history and is peculiar to him. His concurrent life situation, his feelings about the child, and the immediate events of the moment also are factors in the way he behaves. If on occasion he is not the ideally calm, relaxed, unanxious, attentive, judicious, firm but gentle authority, there are good reasons why he is not. Most importantly, he learns from each such experience how his every act is invested with qualities of feeling that influence the efficacy of his efforts at therapeutic intervention.

USE OF PHYSICAL RESTRAINT

Similarly, when it becomes necessary to use physical restraint, the most extreme form of therapeutic intervention, the emotional climate conveyed by the therapist must be clearly therapeutic if the intervention is to be effective. It is not enough that destructive behavior is stopped by evoking fear, for example. Without reducing the motivating conflict, a forced change in the child's behavior is meaningless and often actually dangerous. The child, made angry and rebellious by retaliatory measures, will await his opportunity for revenge with even greater hostile intent than before. On the other hand, even if no change in behavior occurs, a contribution to the reduction of anxiety may be made if the therapist in exercising restraint is relatively free of conflict.

Physical intervention with some children, especially those who are aggressively psychotic, is often the first recognizable technical measure that aborts destructive behavior. With the cessation of hostile and destructive behavior comes some reduction of conflict, since the consequences of such behavior—namely, guilt, fear of retaliation, massive anxiety, and further defiance—fade away when this behavior is curbed. Not only is the disappearance of these distressing feelings relieving in itself, but the possibility of progressive therapeutic work is enhanced. Other contributions to the reduction of the child's internal conflict are the therapist's attitude and manner of exercising physical restraint, his comments, and the alternative modes of expression he offers to the child. These factors help the child to begin to discriminate between the internal conflict and the external reality of the therapeutic situation.

Let us start at a moment when the therapist seizes the wrist of a self-punitive child who is about to slap himself viciously in the face. The child struggles to escape, becomes furiously angry when he cannot, twists in all directions, and hits at the therapist with his free hand. In self-defense the therapist seizes that hand too. Even more furious, the child kicks, and to protect himself, the therapist envelops him with his arms and legs. The child, now impotent to act, strains in fury. If he is not mute, he will shout, curse, and accuse.

Through physical contact with the child, the therapist will learn to distinguish a relaxed muscle tone—one sign that internal conflict has diminished—from a flaccid or melting muscle tone, with the child a dead weight—an indication that a resolution of conflict has not yet been achieved. He will learn also to distinguish firm tone from taut muscle under tension, indicating readiness to spring into impulsive action. These shifts in tone will become clues, telling him when to loosen his grip and or when to resume restraint. Through these and other perceptions the therapist is alerted to prevent destructive behavior and is prepared to allow the fullest possible display of emotion by the child.

In this way the child experiences the nonauthoritarian use of superior strength. Sensing the attitudes and manner with which he is restrained, he learns to discriminate the behavior of the therapist from that of other persons; that is, if the therapist is reasonably free of sadistic or retaliatory feelings, the child experiences restraint that is devoid of revengeful hurt.

The therapist's efforts to verbalize his feelings, concerns, and hunches are important and necessary adjuncts to the effective use of physical restraint. For example, he may, while restraining the child, reaffirm his determination to prevent injury or hurt, or he may voice an idea or impression about what motivated the sudden eruption of violent behavior. On occasion he may express concern about not being more helpful, or even his anger at the patient's having hurt him. His verbalizations are aimed at clarifying, simultaneously for himself and the child, his own feelings, intuitions, and hopes. In all this the child has the opportunity to experience another person, the therapist, living through the welter of his own feelings without acting them out towards the child in any egocentric or sadomasochistic way. Gradually the child may perceive a new solution for his conflicts as he begins to identify with the therapist's reactions and the therapist's strength to restrain his destructive impulses. A sort of confirmatory test for the precision of the therapist's work are those occasions when the child becomes calm and engages in more integrative and satisfying activities. On the other hand, if the child intensifies and prolongs his destructive behavior, a search for causal factors in the counter-transference or in the child's environment is indicated.

The appropriate use of physical restraint can dramatically initiate a process in which the formerly violent release of a turmoil of libidinous feelings, anxiety, and rage through destructive behavior gradually is converted to expression through alternative and less destructive behaviors. When an alternative way of expressing destructive feelings is available through the therapist, the climate becomes more therapeutically relaxed. There is then greater opportunity for resolving conflict and for learning ways to gratify the libidinous impulses which have been warded off. As a result, the intense impulse causing destructive behavior is reduced.

THE THERAPEUTIC VALUE OF CONTROLS

In other words, one individual may control the behavior of another in a way that benefits both. If inner controls are chronically unreliable, as in chronic offenders, the application of consistently reliable controls at critical moments is necessary. Sooner or later these controls are adopted by the offender himself because he learns that they help him to feel better and to live better. Controls from without become converted to controls from within. Thus an important integrated learning experience occurs. The modification in behavior is not the result of fear of consequences, a dubious deterrant; nor does the individual feel coerced. Destructive behavior simply becomes less necessary when it is perceived as a futile effort to escape from the internal turmoil.

Perhaps no one sensed the importance of controls more poignantly than the Hierens boy, of Chicago. Apparently unable to prevent himself from raping and killing, he is reported to have written with lipstick on the wall over the bed of one of his victims, "For heaven's sake catch me before I kill more!"(1). Less dramatic are those instances when a destructive juvenile delinquent is apprehended. At the moment of arrest he may struggle and protest in a way remindful of the restrained child in the playroom. Yet this emotional flare-up ends with confinement, and he becomes as relieved and calm as the child whose destructive play is successfully interrupted. Like the child, the delinquent's emotional conflict and its attendant turmoil is reduced because others have therapeutically contained his destructive behavior when he would not or could not.

One of the complications in the use of controls occurs while they are being exercised. For example, if a child responds to restraint by relaxing after a stormy interval, and if the therapist continues restraint, having failed to notice the change in the child, the child may interpret his behavior as restrictive and punitive. The initial relief and even gratitude brought about by effective controls will disappear almost instantly. Disappointed and hurt, the child will again become resentful and renew his struggles. The therapist may sense only vaguely that something has gone awry, and will be at a loss to know how to quell this new outburst. The tragedy is that now the therapist is involved and a proper, corrective intervention has been converted, by the subtle, unobserved dynamic shift, into one that is needlessly restraining. The therapist's continuing uncertainty prolongs the impasse and results in another defeat for himself and the child.

I am trying to stress what is dynamic in the exercise of controls and to call explicit attention to that climate which is so essential to the efficacy of the process. The actual act of physical intervention is similar to other efforts at control in nonclinical situations, such as verbal admonitions, warnings, or statements of conditions and alternatives. Like all acts, physical interventions are focal manifestations in time, crystallized at certain moments from the flux of human feelings by one individual in response to another. Behavior should adapt promptly to changing conditions, otherwise it quickly becomes static, archaic, useless, and even harmful. The solution to the problem of controls in the playroom lies in our capacity to follow the child; to be aware of our attitudes from moment to moment; to modify our behavior as quickly as our patient alters his; to hold him instantly when indicated; to release him with precise timing; to allow him the widest latitude of behavior within the therapeutic situation; and, at critical times, to say the helpful thing, even frank revelations of our own feelings.

I hope I have not given the impression that a therapist can always provide this perfect, sensitive attention, even in the relatively ideal one-to-one relationship, free from interfering external circumstances, provided by the playroom. Every playroom, with its splattered walls and broken toys, is witness to the contrary. Sometimes the therapist, to avoid risking injury, may restrict the range of the child's activities by removing potentially dangerous toys such as popguns or sharp tools. At certain times and with certain children, he may forbid the use of water, paint, hammers, etc., when reluctant to confront the child with physical restraint. Because of the wide range of their skills and experience, different therapists use established technical procedures differently, or they may create new methods to meet an unprecedented situation.

This, then, is an introduction to the use of controls in the playroom. Because the rules are simple and explicit, and because close supervision is available if needed, a wide latitude of free behavior occurs within nondestructive limits. A community, on the other hand, presents a more complex situation. Its rules—laws, procedures, policies, and definitions of limits and conditions—are administered by agency workers. In the legal field, and probably elsewhere, some of these formulations have punitive provisions, i.e., incarceration, fines, or restrictive requirements. It is sometimes difficult for a correctional worker or a law enforcer to discriminate for himself and for the offender that it is not he who is being punitive; or to express personal reservations about punitive aspects of a law while still enforcing it. In doing this he resembles the therapist in the playroom in that he clearly, concisely, and meaningfully poses alternatives to the offender. Like the therapist, he confronts the offender with his own responsibility to determine consequences for himself—a very therapeutic process, indeed.

The chore of the correctional worker with a client who has stirred up hostility in community agency workers, many of whom look to the correctional worker for solutions, or the job of the law enforcer who encounters a defiant youth in the street, is quite a different matter from controlling a seven-year-old child in the playroom. Nevertheless, as in therapy, many ways are found to solve these problems. They include such things as mobilization of people to provide strength adequate enough to make itself felt, and incarceration, which, like hospitalization, may help to isolate a problem for more definitive treatment and planning.

However, when destructive behavior by a client is perpetuated or aggravated, self-examination by the worker is indicated, in the same manner as a therapist must examine his own countertransference feelings. I am referring to such things as the sense of hopelessness felt by a probation officer towards a probationer who is hostile, provocative, and nonappreciative despite the officer's efforts; the sense of futility he feels when he recognizes that the family influences responsible for the offender's behavior are still operating and are defeating all his efforts; the sense of being at a loss to know how to advise a parent who is similarly at a loss to deal with his delinquent child; the annoyance at the probationer who misses appointments, comes late, and calls insistently for help at the wrong times; the self-blame at a probationer's recidivism; the hesitation to take indicated legal action for fear of spoiling rapport; covertly opposing hierarchal superiors, or differing with them without daring to voice this fact; being subjected to the pressure of newspapers or articulate members of the community; or even being behind in his dictation and summaries, with resulting chronic uneasiness.

However, even the most experienced correctional worker, attempting to help a highly impulsive client, may fail to be effective or will not see results immediately. As in work with very disturbed children, it often takes accumulated and varied experience over a period of time before results become evident, if the behavior of the patient is the sole criterion. While a favorable immediate shift in the patient's behavior conveys useful and hoped for information, with some patients the therapist learns to rely more on how he himself feels when he exercises controls. In time he develops a sense of whether he is acting therapeutically or is becoming personally involved because of his own conflicts. In the latter case, among other clues he may experience lingering uneasiness and dissatisfaction long after his interview with the patient is over; or he may obscure his uneasiness with equally revealing glee and even rationalized boastfulness which hide subtle revengefulness. Such feelings, unpleasant as they may be, are often the beginning of a new learning experience for him. Either he finds that his own feelings and thinking fall into place by themselves, or he resolves them through discussions with his supervisor or other colleagues and, again, knows how to proceed. He may need to discover, over and over again, that the prime criterion of success in professional work is not immediate effectiveness with others, desirable as this goal is, but competence. With it the exercise of authority will sooner or later take on meaning for the patient. And with competence the question of whether controls are therapeutic vanishes. As a matter of fact, in certain circumstances therapy cannot proceed without it.

REFERENCES

1. Kennedy, F., Hoffman, H. R., & Haines, W. H. A study of William Hierens. Am. J. Psychiat., 104: 113-121, 1947.

SECTION THREE

EFFORTS AT PSYCHIATRIC TREATMENT

INTRODUCTION

"Unrewarding" and "discouraging" are perhaps the least negative of the adjectives used to describe the difficulties encountered in the treatment of the antisocial child. The strain on the therapist and the relative lack of effectiveness of therapeutic measures have long been commented on. Perhaps, as August Aichhorn mentioned in Wayward Youth, one should be a cured delinquent to be an effective therapist. Or perhaps, as was indicated in Section Two, one needs to have clarified for oneself the differences between authoritative and authoritarian attitudes.

The role of the family in the treatment of delinquents is a recent consideration. Its problems and the measures required for effective treatment are described in one of the other papers in this section.

SOME IMPRESSIONS FROM CLINICAL EXPERIENCE WITH DELINQUENTS*

S. A. Szurek

Thus every type of delinquency requires a special type of treatment. In all cases, however, the treatment must concern itself with the further development of the ego-ideal, and we must put the question thus: how can we direct social retraining in order to bring about corrections of character in the individual? (1)

It is well known to those psychiatric clinicians who deal with children that the term "delinquency" is both overly broad in its implications and lacking in precision—a fault that often characterizes psychiatric terms and concepts. "Delinquency"—in a psychiatric sense—includes a large variety of personality structures and of persistent patterns of interpersonal behavior, which are the result of different combinations of constitutional and social determinants. In its widest sense, the term "delinquency" refers to a child's or adolescent's failure to conform to generally accepted standards of behavior, or to a positive rebellion against those standards. Such a child usually does not manifest any obvious evidence of associated mental or somatic disorders. It is not the purpose of this paper to delineate the complex symptomatic factors of delinquency. We are all familiar with the varieties of maldevelopment of character, the failures of personality integration, the various constellations of family and social settings, and the types of life histories which are or may be included in this concept of delinquency. Let us leave the conception in all its vagueness and assume some understanding of the general field of human behavior it implies.

---

*Reprinted with permission from Searchlights on Delinquency, K. R. Eissler, ed. International Universities Press, New York, 1949, pp. 115-127.

One useful contribution to this discussion would be a summary of personal, professional experiences with delinquents. Therefore I offer here a few specific examples of such experiences, with some general remarks and impressions drawn from almost a decade of participation in the work of psychiatric clinics and hospital wards for children.

A well-dressed, rather handsome boy of sixteen was brought to the clinic by his distraught father because he had several times forged the name of the father's former employer to checks which he cashed. In his interview with the clinic psychiatrist the boy was quite at ease, frankly answering questions about himself, his family, and the reasons for his being brought to the clinic. There was no marked evidence of guilt or anxiety when he acknowledged that he had committed the forgeries, that in the past he had had other encounters with the police for stealing, and that he did not like to go to school. He could not say he had any definite ambitions, but he "had thought of" joining the Marines. He gave other facts about his past, without lengthy elaboration, seeming indifferent and almost bored. Shrugging his shoulders, he said he did not know why he forged the checks: he just needed more money for dates and fun because his father had recently taken a position less lucrative than selling automobiles. He returned to the waiting room after the interview and slumped indolently behind a magazine.

The father in his interview, on the other hand, tensely poured out his story with little need for encouragement or questions. He was utterly baffled by his son's acts and did not know what he should do. After his torrent of speech subsided, gradual questioning elicited the information of which the following is but a brief summary. (The whole affair had made the mother too sick and nervous—as she was so often—to be able to come to the clinic.)

The mother had been eager to have a daughter but had had three miscarriages in the first few years of their marriage. To assuage her extreme disappointment during her recovery from the last of these miscarriages, the father went to a private adoption agency and brought her a child—the son who was to become our patient. Within the next few years they adopted a daughter and finally a boy was born to them. The mother was often dissatisfied with her husband for his lack of enthusiasm for her preferred recreations, especially dancing. The older son had always been a problem because of his association with bad companions, his truancy from school, and his stealing. Yet the father liked the boy, perhaps because he himself had been rather "wild" in his youth and had run away from home to join the Marines at sixteen by falsifying his age. He had made a good record in his two "hitches" in the service and had brought up his son "on the Marines."

Some six months before their visit to the clinic, after the father had been forced to take a job as a guard in a defense plant, the boy had announced that he would like to leave school and go to work. Somewhat reluctantly his parents agreed. Weeks went by, and although he had made some efforts, the boy was still without a job. The father became impatient and finally insisted on dictating a letter of application for several jobs advertised in the want ads. The boy soon had a job but was discharged after one week. Two weeks before the visit to the clinic the father was notified by his former employer that several checks amounting to forty-five dollars had been forged and cashed. The evidence pointed to his son—who admitted it. In a serious effort to impress the boy with the gravity of his offense, the father demanded that the son sign three legal-looking documents. He told his son that one of these would be sent to the bank, another to the employer, and the third to the judge. If there were any repetitions of forgery, the son would thereby be automatically remanded to the authorities. The son signed the documents. A week later he forged another check for fifteen dollars. The father then became desperate and, upon the advice of friends, brought the boy to the clinic.

In the ensuing discussion it became evident to both the father and the psychiatrist that by the last forgery the boy had called his father's bluff. The father felt "licked" and helpless. He had thought of permitting the boy to join the Marines but was afraid the boy would damage his father's reputation in this branch of the service. He asked pleadingly for advice or suggestions. At this impasse the psychiatrist wondered whether there was anything left to do except for the father frankly to admit to the boy that he felt helpless, bewildered, and defeated. The father anxiously asked whether he should do this, to which the psychiatrist replied he could not urge or advise any course of action upon the father which he himself did not feel he wanted or could undertake. It seemed to the psychiatrist that since the boy had checkmated his father; since the father had done everything except treat his son like the man he wanted him to become; since he had not been able to admit his defeat to his son— the next move obviously seemed to be up to the boy. Perhaps the father could ask his son what he wanted to do. Seemingly eased by the discussion, the father suddenly decided this was all he could do and that he would do it.

A week later the father returned to the clinic alone, looking much happier, and enthusiastically reported the events of the week. On the way home from the previous clinic visit, father and son had had the most serious conversation they had ever had, during which both were deeply moved. The boy had wept a little and suddenly announced he was going to get a job. A day later he was at work and seemed a changed person. He was too busy to come to the clinic again, and his father thought further visits by either his son or himself were unnecessary. The father said he felt as if a tremendous load had been lifted from his shoulders; he was very grateful and promised he would return if difficulties even began to appear. Because the psychiatrist soon left the clinic for military service, it was impossible to follow up this father and son story.

On another occasion the clinic psychiatrist was consulted by a young male social worker (a member of the staff of a denominational welfare agency of the city) regarding a sixteen-year-old boy. The boy had appeared at the juvenile court repeatedly following episodes of disappearance from home, truancy, and burglary. The court had almost decided to commit the boy to the state reformatory when the agency, anxious to keep children of its denomination out of the reformatory, urgently requested that the court grant the boy probation under the agency's guardianship. Since the boy appeared to be a doubtful prospect—both because of his longstanding indifference to his family and because of his family's sense of resignation and defeat, if not indifference, toward him—the social worker asked the psychiatrist what help the clinic could offer. Could a staff member arrange to give the boy psychotherapeutic interviews?

The psychiatrist, recalling his many failures in attempts at direct psychotherapy with adolescents of this sort from just such homes as this one, was dubious: such boys rarely responded to psychotherapeutic interviews. They rarely seemed troubled or under any inner stress. They had little to say and acted as if they were more interested in doing things and having fun instead of "just talking" to a psychiatrist. Occasionally, if they became attached to the therapist and continued their visits to the clinic for more than a few weeks, they began insistently to demand that he intercede with the agency, their parents, or school authorities to secure for them more money, privileges, gifts, or special changes of curriculum. They might come late or at odd hours for their appointments, or ask to ride in the psychiatrist's car or to be allowed to see him at his home on weekends. The slightest disappointment of these wishes, no matter how unreasonable, often prompted them to discontinue their clinic visits; it was frequently followed by some delinquent act. Because of such experiences, the psychiatrist told the worker he was doubtful of the value of psychotherapeutic interviews in such a case.

However, the psychiatrist had been impressed with the fruitful results of the short, weekly recreation trips on which the clinic's social workers had taken several moderately impulsive preadolescent or adolescent children of the same sex as the worker. During such trips the workers made no suggestions that the child discuss his problems, but accepted such confidences as were spontaneously offered during the trip. He asked the agency worker whether, since he would be responsible for finding a foster home and a school placement for the boy and would be supplying his spending money, he would also be willing and able to find the time to work with this impulsive youth. The psychiatrist offered to be available for regular consultation. The social worker hesitantly agreed and asked what should be his general attitude toward the boy.

It was decided that, above all, the worker would be as honest as possible with the boy about everything. This would include not only re-emphasis of the fact that this was the boy's last chance to stay out of a reformatory; that in the event of another offense neither the court nor the agency could again intercede for him, nor would they feel justified in doing so. It would also be necessary to make it quite clear that the social worker, although willing to do all he could, doubted that he could immediately satisfy all the boy's needs and wishes; that he even doubted whether the boy and he could really "hit it off" together and eventually trust each other. Knowing that the boy had for many years felt distrustful of anyone's sincerity towards him and had impatiently done what he could to satisfy his impulses himself, the social worker thought that there was little chance the boy could restrain himself long enough to give either of them time to learn whether things could be different. With neither person having reason for trust at the outset, the social worker was frankly skeptical of the chance for success in their joint venture—but he was willing to try.

This was somewhat against the social worker's principle of not using "threats" with children. But he nevertheless agreed that only frankness about the boy's social reality and about the psychological reality between himself and the boy promised an atmosphere in which he—and therefore perhaps the boy—could begin their relationship.

There followed an eighteen-month period of fruitful collaboration between the social worker and the psychiatrist. The social worker found a home—in fact, a succession of them—for the boy. He provided him with spending money and went with him on a number of occasions for various forms of recreation. He made himself available to the boy at his office or on the phone as his time permitted. He listened to the boy's requests considerately, granting those within his power and regretfully denying others. Several school placements, despite conferences between the worker and school counselors, were such failures (because of the boy's poor achievement and truancies) that it was decided to let him go to work. Within a year after he began working, the boy had found a job as a messenger for a firm and was carrying over $10,000 at a time to the bank. Eventually there was—undirected by the social worker—a gradual rapprochement between the boy and his family, and he finally returned to live with them.

The social worker and the psychiatrist—who never saw the boy—met weekly at first, to discuss progress and the details of the social worker's experience with the boy. Later conferences were less and less frequent. Occasionally there were discussions between them by telephone, especially during crises. In these conferences it became clear that the social worker had come to feel a good deal of spontaneous warmth and admiration for some of the qualities of the boy's personality.

As the rapport between the social worker and the psychiatrist increased, the former mentioned that he could understand some of the boy's feelings toward adults in authority because of his own memories of adolescent experiences. Even though this empathy between the social worker and the boy (which early showed itself in a degree of frankness and directness on the part of the boy, often surprising to the worker) was the basis for the generally favorable direction of the boy's readjustment, it was also the source of some difficulties and crises. Following several occasions on which the boy failed to carry out a mutually agreed-upon course of action, consultation with the psychiatrist uncovered the fact that the social worker had had some inner doubts or uneasiness regarding the matter discussed with the boy. For one reason or another—often because he was not clearly aware of his own conflict—the social worker had not voiced his divided feelings to the boy. Almost inevitably a failure or crisis in the boy's adjustment followed.

The social worker finally became convinced that the boy at such times responded in terms of the worker's own unspoken and unacknowledged feelings toward the boy, and nothing less than the full expression of the social worker's attitudes would help the boy to choose the path leading to his own best self-interest. This meant telling the boy, whenever the social worker felt it, that he was angry with, disappointed in, or regretful of, the boy's behavior or impulses. At times it meant admitting that he was skeptical of the truth of some story the boy told; or that he felt some admiration for the boy's rebelliousness, even though he knew he should demand that the boy submit and conform. It meant admitting to the boy that his pride was involved in "succeeding" with him, even though he knew that the boy might prefer to do something other than what the worker thought "best" for him. Finally, it meant telling him quite frankly whenever the boy made him feel worried, uneasy, or fright-

ened. The worker thus learned that when he could say some of
these things out loud to the boy, he felt easier and more able to
consider the boy's impulses from the boy's point of view; and the
result was that the boy usually responded in a way which allayed
the tensions in both of them.

Unfortunately, here too circumstances prevented a follow-up to
learn of this boy's eventual adjustment to life. It is probably too
much to expect that such a relatively short period of work could be
decisive for the later life of a boy with such character structure
and disturbed family relations. However, the experience was an
illuminating one for both the psychiatrist and the worker.

PROBLEMS OF THERAPY

Other clinical experiences have suggested the importance of a
very flexible approach. This is especially true with children or
adolescents whose relations with other persons are characterized
by impulsive self-gratification; by inadequate restraint of sexual,
revengeful, or exploitative impulses; or by poorly integrated loy-
alties and interests. The factor of major importance in determining the choice of therapeutic effort may be the presence or
absence of some degree of parental affection and warmth in the
child's life. One is tempted to assert that, other things being equal,
the less the child has experienced an essential and spontaneous interest in his welfare and wishes, the more difficult will be the
therapeutic problem. However ambivalently his natural or adoptive
parents may feel toward him, the treatment of such a child will still
be less difficult than that of one who has had no parents. Often the
parentless child has experienced numerous failures in foster home
placement before the clinician is consulted, and the agency responsible for the child is uncertain of being able to find a home in which
the child is likely to succeed.

If such a child is less than ten years old, the agency often insistently requests that we attempt treatment within a psychiatric hospital ward for children or some other residential treatment center
before they try to place him in a foster home. If we grant such a
request, the hospital staff encounters difficulties because the
child's demands divert their time and emotional resources from
the more inhibited psychoneurotic and psychotic children. The
impulsive and neglected orphan, if thwarted in even minor ways,
promptly responds with hostile destructiveness and agressiveness
and directs his response in various individual ways. He may make
use of children whom he has intimidated; he may weld the other
children into "gangs" allied against the personnel or weaker children, or he may be destructive of hospital property. His insatiable

demands for affection and for durable security are more difficult to meet than those of other children whose parents visit them and give them at least some semblance of belonging to a family.

Placement of such parentless, impulsive children in other public institutions, such as juvenile detention homes, is usually only temporary. This is fortunate, for the prolonged residence enabled by state funds is undesirable: there are few provisions for education or recreation, and too small a staff for the number of children admitted. Such staffs are perforce often, and perhaps in spite of themselves, more apt to be repressive and punitive in attitude than guided by any rational therapeutic principles. Impulsive adolescents, after discharge from these state schools, frequently present problems to their parole officers, who then in turn consult the clinic staff about the inevitable crises which arise when they try to restore them to community life in foster homes. If the parole officer is not overburdened with a large case load, and if the clinic staff has the time, it may be possible to help the officer. Such help is more often fruitful if it is offered by way of conferences regarding his contact and work with the adolescent and his foster parents, than by direct psychotherapy of the adolescent in clinic interview sessions.

Both psychiatrists attached to juvenile court clinics and parole officers sometimes hold misconceptions about the prospects and possibilities of direct psychotherapy in the outpatient clinic. Few in either group appreciate the difficulties involved in the hospital care of impulsively aggressive children or adolescents. Parole officers commonly overestimate the effectiveness of psychiatric treatment—specifically of psychotherapy. Such overestimation may be in part a product of their own deep sense of helplessness in regard to their professional burdens and problems. However, psychiatrists themselves at times increase this overestimation by implied and unrealistic promises of the results of psychotherapy. There is also, of course, the opposite and older attitude among parole officers: namely, skepticism regarding the value of any psychiatric treatment, which may be based on insufficient knowledge or may stem from repeated disappointments.

In their strong desire to keep a particular child—often a young, attractive, and likable youngster—out of public institutions, both parole officers and court psychiatrists may minimize the difficulties of hospital treatment. In these situations their pressure upon the psychiatric clinic to assume the responsibility may stem from several origins. Aside from whatever personal feelings they may have developed for the particular child, they are often fully aware of the gross inadequacies both of their own residences and services and of those of the state institutions.

Court psychiatrists also are occasionally prone to these misconceptions about treatment because their inadequate clinical experience with this category of psychopathology makes them unable to make a correct diagnosis. Now and then a child is seen at court who seems "anxious" to them, when actually he is thoroughly frightened of the possible consequences of his behavior. This "anxiety," when studied in a psychiatric clinic, shows itself to be not so much genuine anxiety arising from an internalized conscience or superego as fear of the external, impending punishment for transgressions. The child only deepens diagnostic errors if, when asked for the reasons for his behavior, he persistently denies any knowledge or awareness of his motivation. Since he often is not fully aware of them or in his frightened state is unable to state those about which he is clear, he may mislead a relatively inexperienced examiner. The examiner then concludes that such "unconscious" motivation is sufficient indication for dynamic psychotherapy.

Inexperienced psychiatrists may be further misled by statements in the literature regarding the psychodynamics of the neurotic character which they may take to imply that a dynamic or psychoanalytic treatment has been or can be successful. They overlook the fact that the staffs of psychiatric clinics for children rarely have enough therapists who are fully qualified to give psychoanalytic treatment. Even if there were more, qualified therapists, we would be doubtful of their value in these cases for two reasons: first, few therapists or patients would have the time to meet for the frequent therapeutic sessions which classical child analysis requires; and second, we are doubtful that psychotherapy, whether by the play or the interview method, is an effective approach in these cases. The psychotherapeutic method seems to us to be contraindicated for several reasons. In general psychotherapy aims to reverse the psychoneurotic process of repression, and it is devised for this purpose. Its goal is to aid in transforming and integrating the repressed impulses into ego attitudes which are in harmony with such self-esteem as the patient has already integrated. But the impulsive child, in contrast to the psychoneurotically inhibited patient, suffers from lack of restraint of his impulses.

THE IMPORTANCE OF SURROGATE PARENTS

We believe that the impulsive child needs to receive the experience of love previously denied him. He needs the spontaneous, ungrudging warmth of an adult, given to him as a person and not merely as a reward for conformity. He needs this love for the prolonged period necessary for him to develop an essential sense of security. He also needs frank, unyielding firmness coupled with uncompromising fairness and justice. The therapist needs to be able to recognize the many forms which the patient's distrustful, unmodified egocentricity and revengefulness may take, and yet not be swayed from his therapeutic goal. It is extremely difficult—at times impossible—to consistently maintain such attitudes. However, at least an approximation of these conditions may offer a chance that the child will become attached to the adult; if the relationship is continued long enough, he will begin to identify with the adult's ideals, to understand the adult's wishes for his own welfare, and to acquire a new sense of his own worth as a person. In short, he may be able to integrate the beginnings of a new self-respect, of a conscience or more conscience, and of more self-restraint. At the same time the basis of his egocentricity, his distrustful impulsiveness, and his revengefulness may be gradually liquidated as new experiences counteract his former experiences with people.

Aichhorn clearly elucidated this point when he wrote:

Our work differs from that of the psychoanalyst in that we use the transference to accomplish an entirely different task.... In remedial training we cannot be content with transient results which arise from the emotional tie of the dissocial boy or girl to the worker. We must succeed, as in psychoanalysis, in bringing the wayward youth under the influence of the transference to a definite achievement. This achievement consists in a real character change, in the setting up of a socially directed ego ideal, that is, in the retrieving of that part of his development which is necessary for a proper adjustment to society [1, pp. 235-36].

These goals require not only adequate financial support but also—and this is even more necessary—parental substitutes (either in our institutions or outside of them) who have at least some of the qualities described above. Only such parental surrogates may be able to give the time and feeling requisite to redress the balance. Some selected cases may, in addition, need direct psychotherapeutic treatment at the clinic, and the parental surrogate may require concomitant help for his own conflicts during the inevitable times of crisis. In many other instances it may be feasible to have the parole officer or the child placement agency social worker give the foster mother the support and advice she needs, and then to have this agent in turn be briefed by the psychiatrist in regular conferences at the clinic. In an institution the parental surrogate (in the person of matron, cottage father, nurse, or attendant) might similarly benefit from regular discussions with a dynamically oriented and trained psychiatrist about his particular difficulties with a given child. "Forced psychotherapy" with the child may also prove to be an important technical addition whenever there are sufficient psychiatric personnel adequately trained for the peculiarities of this type of psychotherapy (2).

THERAPY WITH NATURAL PARENTS

It should now be clear that the writer considers it imperative to treat the natural parents of an impulsive child when they remain part of the family situation. Their treatment should be as clinically adequate and therapeutically oriented as that given to the child, and treatment of child and parents should be conducted simultaneously. So great is the importance of treating or dealing with the parents that its adequate discussion would require much more space than is here available. A very few comments must suffice.

Our theories of delinquency rest on the implicit assumption—supported by our clinical experience—that the child has failed in certain essential areas of personality integration. He has not integrated into his ego-organization an attitude of confidence that, by and large, his essential needs will be gratified, so he is driven instead to defiant (either openly or surreptitiously), aggressive, and egocentric pursuit of these gratifications. The emphasis is, of course, on the egocentric nature of the pursuit, i.e., its disregard for the rights, needs, or feelings of others. This outcome can occur, according to our hypothesis, only if the child's earliest experiences at the hands of others were similarly without regard for his needs, feelings, or welfare. Such mishandling of the child may stem from a variety of parental attitudes. There may be graded differences of attitudes by one or both parents toward particular aspects of the child's behavior, or one or both parents may have serious conflicts—internal, interpersonal, or in regard to the child—but all of these difficulties have a similar end effect on the child. Moreover, psychotherapy with the parents will be effective only if their conflicts produce in them inner suffering and anxiety. Only by offering the parents psychotherapeutic help in solving their own conflicts will the child's welfare eventually profit. In other words, it is essential for both the parents and the therapist to be aware that the work is not carried on merely for the sake of the child.

Admittedly, persuading such parents to accept therapeutic assistance for their own internal conflicts is often the crucial difficulty[1]. During a crisis, under pressure from police or juvenile court authorities for some delinquent act by their child, parents may be so chagrinned by the threat of social ostracism that genuine anxiety and guilt can be mobilized sufficiently that one or both may be willing to participate in clinical work. Such participation means, ideally, separate therapists for the parent and the child. Occasionally, such parents do seek clinical assistance before the child has actually been arrested, driven perhaps by their own anxieties over early indications of his rebelliousness. In these instances the prognosis for successful therapy is likely to be the best—but such family situations are rare among those most frequently seen in juvenile courts. When parents show relatively less anxiety about their status and self-esteem, and perhaps more resignation or indifference with regard to the child and his behavior, the prognosis for even beginning therapy is rather poor. In these cases the difficulties of treatment approach those common to cases of parentless children.

In the more favorable instances, in which parental anxieties are high, the therapeutic plan may vary from direct treatment of both parents and the child by separate therapists, through treatment of the child and one parent (the more available and emotionally involved parent is preferred), to therapeutic effort with one parent only. It sometimes happens that after work is begun with one parent and the child, the anxieties of the other parent lead him to request help as well. It is natural to ask whether the treatment of only one parent is not adult rather than child psychiatry, especially when the child, having been seen only briefly at the beginning, drops out of treatment because of, or without, improvement. This is a matter of definition depending on the nature of the psychopathology within the family. It becomes difficult to define only if one adheres too rigidly to administration or specialty classifications instead of following the clinical indications of the "problem in nature."

In conclusion, the writer is tempted to condense and oversimplify his clinical experiences (with children who have parents) into a dictum: "The psychoneurotic parent is likely to rear at least one psychopathic child." Some of the factors or variables and their

---

[1]For further elaboration of these difficulties, see Szurek, S. A., Some principles of child guidance practice. Newsletter of the Amer. Assn. of Psychiatric Social Workers, 16:119-20, 1947.

quantitative interrelation which are necessary to produce the psychopathic child have been discussed in Chapter 1. The writer has been impressed with the fact that the ordinal position of the child's birth (e.g., a middle child coming soon after the first-born, or the youngest child coming late after the older siblings) in conjunction with the emotional state of the parents (perhaps more often of the mother), may be an essential determinant of psychopathology. Additional factors which come readily to mind are the sex of the child or his physical qualities, such as resemblance to someone else, which may arouse, intensify, or redirect ancient conflicts between the parents, focusing them toward that particular child. In any case, the content of this dictum may also be stated in a more generalized form: "The most overt symptom of a parental personality disorder is the behavior of his child."

Where a natural parent shows such a personality disorder (and in the writer's experience this occurs frequently, if not invariably), the plan of treatment is determined by the availability of adequate psychotherapeutic skills. In view of the fact that impulsive children and adolescents are, however, ambivalently attached to, and emotionally as well as economically dependent upon, their parents, therapeutic work with the parents is often the most direct approach and most economical use of the clinician's time in solving the problems of the child. Nonetheless, this does not in every case exclude the careful evaluation of the child's accessibility to psychotherapy, or even the offering of such direct treatment as a means toward evaluation. Once again we wish to emphasize the advantages of concomitant therapeutic effort with the parent to assist him in the resolution of the conflicts which were etiologically important in the child's personality problem.

Another important factor which determines the success of clinical efforts was not touched upon in this discussion, namely, the personality of the child's therapist. It is extremely important for the development of empathy and rapport with such aggressive children that the therapist's attitude be infused with elements arising perhaps from his own early experiences which he has resolved and integrated, but which are not unlike those of the impulsive child. In this, too, Aichhorn was clear and emphatic when he wrote:

> I cannot close this book without once more stressing the great importance of the personality of the workers in this field. You have seen that a character change in the delinquent means a change in his ego ideal. This occurs when new traits are taken over by the individual. The source of these traits is the worker. He is the important object with whom the dissocial child or youth can retrieve the defective

or non-existent identification and with whom he can experience all the things in which his father failed him. With the worker's help, the youth acquires the necessary feeling relation to his companions which enables him to overcome the dissocial traits. The word "father-substitute," so often used in connection with remedial education, receives its rightful connotation in this conception of the task.

What helps the worker most in therapy with the dissocial? The transference! And especially what we recognize as the positive transference. It is above all the tender feeling for the teacher that gives the pupil the incentive to do what is prescribed and not to do what is forbidden. The teacher, as a libidinally charged object for the pupil, offers traits for identification that bring about a lasting change in the structure of the ego ideal. This in turn effects a change in the behavior of the formerly dissocial child. We cannot imagine a person who is unsocial as a worker in this field. We assume therefore that the ego ideal of the child will be corrected through the worker's help in bringing him to a recognition of the claims of society and to participation in society [1, pp. 234-35].

REFERENCES

1. AICHHORN, A. Wayward youth. New York: Viking Press, 1935.

2. WHITAKER, C. Ormsby Village: An experiment with forced psychotherapy in the rehabilitation of the delinquent adolescent. Psychiatry, 9:239-250, 1946.

THE ROLE OF CLINICIANS IN THE TREATMENT
OF JUVENILE DELINQUENTS*

S. A. Szurek

Delinquent behavior is essentially that behavior which does not conform to the rules of interpersonal relations accepted by a community. It is defined by the attitudes held by both the delinquent and the community with respect to property rights, sexual behavior, school attendance, and especially expressions of hostile and destructive impulses.

Delinquent behavior presents to those who would understand it a complex problem in human motivation. Both the social sciences (anthropology, sociology, psychology, and economics,) and medical sciences (especially psychiatry,) are concerned in its solution. Although it is an oversimplification, one may divide delinquent children and youth into two classes: first, those in whom there is primarily a psychopathological distortion of personality organization, and, second, those whose behavior is predominantly determined by social-cultural frustrations deriving from the family, the neighborhood, or the gang. Almost always both factors are involved, and no particular delinquent child will fall neatly into either class. The cultural frustrations of the parents are likely to affect their discipline of their child, and their cultural status is often an important factor in determining the child's attitudes toward their authority and precepts.

Because of the uniqueness of each individual delinquent, clinical study is the only method by which a rational plan for treatment can be formulated. By clinical study one means the collection of pertinent biographical data, a physical examination, an assessment of intellectual and personality assets and liabilities, as well as a close scrutiny of the cultural milieu of the delinquent (9). From these data the experienced clinician—or a collaborating group of specialists—is better able to estimate the processes which brought about

*Reprinted with permission from Federal Probation, 7:30-33, 1943.

the delinquency and to reach a decision on the course of treatment. However, even if the clinician perfectly appraises the situation, he still may be in the position of the astronomer who can foresee a celestial cataclysm but is helpless to avert it.

TREATMENT OF NEUROTIC AND CHARACTER DISORDERS

Division of delinquents into those with predominantly psycho-pathological personalities and those who are relatively well integrated with _some_ group, permits some practical planning for treatment. The Gluecks (1), Healy (3), and many others have emphasized repeatedly the distinction between these two groups. The consensus is that those youths who come into conflict with the dominant mores of their culture chiefly because of disorders in personality development represent a minority of delinquents. Of this minority a large proportion manifests personality traits which in adulthood will be easily recognizable to the experienced psychiatrist as those syndromes variously called psychopathic personalities, "moral imbeciles," or neurotic characters. The remainder of those with psychopathological tendencies may be classified as having psychoneurotic disorders. There is a narrow line between these two clinical syndromes, but it is generally conceded that treatment of the extreme case of psychopathic personality is as yet an unsolved clinical problem. With respect to treatment, two points must be emphasized: first, prolonged therapy is essential for the alleviation of psychoneurotic disorders; and second, therapy must include the whole family—especially the parent emotionally more important to the child—and not just the young patient himself.

The clinical experience of psychotherapists in the last two or three decades has established beyond any doubt that for any measurable degree of cure of psychoneurotic disorders a prolonged and rather intensive therapy by adequately trained psychiatrists is essential. Obviously there are different degrees of illness and the length and intensiveness of a 12- or 24-month period of analytic treatment—even if it were available—may not be essential for some relief of symptoms. Nevertheless, it is indubitable that analytic training, or some equivalent, in treatment of psychoneuroses is the best equipment for a psychiatrist who is forced to offer treatment on a much reduced scale in terms of its duration and the frequency of interviews. This training is expensive, lengthy, and frequently difficult to obtain. The question of the time necessary for treatment is one which well could occupy all of the space allotted for this discussion; but it must suffice to say that if there were adequate appreciation of this fact, many misunderstandings now current would disappear.

The second point, the need to treat psychotherapeutically the parent or parents of the neurotically disturbed child in addition to offering direct treatment to the child (4,5,6,7,8) is also one which requires more emphasis and elaboration than space permits. It is possible only to refer to the fact that clinicians with wide experience in child psychiatry are clearly aware that the neurotic anxiety underlying the symptoms in the child have their chief genesis in some emotional disorder of the adults upon whom the child depends. It has become evident that without some amelioration of the parental anxieties and insecurities about the child, direct therapy of the child is less successful both in extent and in the time required to achieve relief of symptoms. The most pertinent aspect of this question is the fact that giving to a parent who is deeply in conflict simple advice and suggestions for managing a child's behavior is generally futile. Such parents have usually done all they emotionally have been able to do, have listened to many advisers and tried without a sense of conviction, and certainly without success, many measures before they reach the clinic.

Concerning the treatment of the child or adolescent manifesting that peculiar aggressive instability, that distortion of the conscience which we clinically term "psychopathic personality trends" or "neurotic character traits," it may be added that there are indications that only if treatment of the situation is possible early enough in the child's life and for a long enough period of time, is there some hope of averting serious disorders of character (5). For these conditions neither the mental hospital nor the penal institution afford any appreciable degree of cure. One emphasizes treatment of the situation because here again parental attitudes need to be fundamentally modified, even perhaps to the point of permitting placement of the child in an appropriate school, institution, or another home. Otherwise, the problem presented by such a child in adolescence remains in large part unsolved because of lack of appropriate institutional facilities staffed with really competent personnel, as well as lack of adequate legal instrumentality to make such treatment possible. Prone as these individuals are to disturbances of psychotic-like intensity while confined in the prison and yet not durably disordered as are the true psychotics, they are likely to be discharged from the mental hospital as "without psychosis" although they actually have shown evidence of psychosis in the prison.

The majority of delinquent youth are relatively well integrated in personality structure and development. These are the children and adolescents who have lasting, genuine friendships with playmates or gang, and who manifest loyalty and concern for the welfare of their parents, siblings, and friends. They are relatively secure within themselves. Various degrees of real economic or social frustrations for their families, neighborhoods, or social stratum contribute to individual discontents which, when combined, lead to delinquent group behavior. By individual discontents one refers to such disintegrating experiences, in infancy or early childhood, in the relations within the family, especially with the parents, as are peculiar and unique to the youth among his siblings. The conscience of this type of delinquent youth, though well developed in the ethics of his group, does not include restraints against offenses directed toward the larger world in which they live. Delinquency may pay off in lucrative return from adults as well as in greater prestige in the gang. The child's realization of his parents' lack of prestige and status, because of their cultural inadequacies, often contributes to the decrease or loss of parental ability to give adequate supervision in those instances where parental attitudes reflect the mores of the larger community.

The end result of childhood frustrations may be the inculcation of deeply ingrained attitudes of suspicion and general hostility to any representatives of the larger world. The teacher, the judge, the probation officer, and the staff of the psychiatric clinic, become the legitimate objects of deception, evasion, surreptitious defiance, or overt hostile acts if opportunities present themselves. They, and the house-fathers, teachers, and disciplinarians at training schools and reformatories, have the added burden of overcoming such obstacles within the child's feelings before the delinquent child can begin to experience any confidence that the larger world is not too hostile and too depriving, but is instead a place in which he can live in relative peace and collaboration. It is only after a long period in which the child really experiences a chance to obtain satisfactions of his legitimate needs for security, prestige, and warmth in an atmosphere of firm but tolerant justice, that his earlier attitudes of hostile cynicism toward the mores of his community may begin to change.

This sketchy review of a large subject may afford some basis for understanding the principles upon which clinicians operate. It may permit a glimpse of the reasons why single, brief, clinical examination is inadequate to deal with these complicated processes and why the emphasis of clinicians is on a treatment program and its possibilities. It now may be somewhat clearer why clinicians repeatedly emphasize that the essential need is to deal by individual casework techniques with the entire family of the younger children who have been called (perhaps somewhat optimistically) predelinquents, before they have become old enough and strong enough to come into conflict with people on that larger stage of life outside the inner family circle or the classroom and schoolyard.

One includes in casework techniques mobilization of all community resources to supply economic, recreational, and health needs. With limited facilities in all communities—and a total lack of them in many—to administer casework service by adequately trained and adequately paid social workers, the examining clinicians, although seeing the problems fairly clearly and recognizing the need for prolonged and adequate help, become aware of the similarity of their position to that of the aforementioned astronomer.

To summarize, the techniques are known, their relative utility is fairly accurately recognized, but the demand for service is overwhelming. Limited chiefly by the time available to examining procedures, without being able to institute and supervise or collaborate in adequate treatment programs, the clinicians are not surprised at the dissatisfaction, disappointment, and often derogation of their efforts. Pressed by insistent demands of both sides—the injured parties and the family of the delinquent—the teacher, the judge, and probation officer often turn to the clinician with an unconscious wish for a magical resolution of the aroused hostile tensions of the adults involved and for securing the patent needs of the child. The suggestions for treatment offered by the clinic staff not infrequently are more or less frankly regarded as a kind of "mollycoddling," especially when the court's facilities reflecting those of the community are also limited.

THE ROLE OF THE CLINICIAN IN RELATION TO THE PROBATION OFFICER AND THE CASEWORKER

The role of the clinician in relation to the probation officers and caseworkers—especially when these are male workers assigned to preadolescent and adolescent delinquent boys—is conceived to be that of consultant and supervisor. Since the anxiety of the nonpsychopathic delinquent is due more to the threat of punishment (i.e., incarceration, discipline in the training school) by external authority than to an overactive conscience as in the psychoneurotic individual, direct psychotherapeutic efforts of the psychiatrist with the child in the interview situation cannot be expected to be of much utility. Some clinical experience, however, suggests that when the probation officer or male worker allows a relationship with the child to develop on the basis of recreational trips, or on the basis of other real needs of the child, without any attempt at a pseudo-psychiatric probing into the child's feelings, repeated consultation with a psychiatrist is of great value to the progress of therapy. By virtue of his training and experience in interpersonal dynamics the psychiatrist can and does help the worker understand more clearly the meaning of the child's attitudes toward the worker. The sharing of the clinical responsibility is also of considerable value. The success of such collaboration between the caseworker and the psychiatrist depends in a large measure upon the degree of professional training and experience of the worker. Other factors such as a reasonable caseload, adequate compensation, security of tenure, as well as well-integrated personality, are obviously of considerable importance in assuring in the worker a mature, tolerant firmness toward the child's suspicions and inevitably provocative hostility. It is this need for a rational, nonretaliatory attitude and frequently an almost infinite patience in such treatment that makes the average nonprofessional individual less useful. Dependent as he is for his almost entire satisfaction upon some grateful or affectionate response from the child for what is usually a charitable or spare-time effort, it is not surprising that impatient, and often unconscious hostile and irrational reactions of the nonprofessional to the child make for early termination of any relationship which can be useful to the child. The extreme readiness to hostile responses on the part of the child, both direct and disguised, also makes it almost imperative that psychiatric supervision be provided.

Plans for an integrated program of treatment within a training school, with adequate supervision of the child in the community following discharge, need to be worked out carefully. Essential to the success of the program are: careful selection of adequately trained, mature personnel, with adequate compensation and security of tenure; programs to train the children for occupations that really exist in the community; sufficient recreational facilities and funds; and, the marshalling of the community resources to provide adequate homes, further education, or employment. Real power in the hands of the supervising parole officer to return the delinquent to the school if necessary, coupled with a genuine interest in providing the youth with real security and satisfactions in his community, also seem elementary essentials in increasing the percentage of successful adjustments. Psychiatric consultation and supervision of the caseworker's efforts throughout the various stages of treatment—prior to and during, as well as after, the residence in the school—are to the staff of a clinic rather important ingredients of the prescription.

REFERENCES

1. GLUECK, S., & GLUECK, E. T. One thousand juvenile delinquents. Cambridge: Harvard University Press, 1934.

2. GREIG, A. B. The problem of the parent in child analysis. Psychiatry 3:539-543, 1940.

3. HEALY, W., & BRONNER, A. F. New light on delinquency and its treatment. New Haven: Yale University Press, 1937.

4. JOHNSON, A. M., FALSTEIN, E. I., SZUREK, S. A., & SVENDSEN, M. School phobia. Amer. J. Orthopsychiat. 11:702-711, 1941. Reprinted in I. N. Berlin & S. A. Szurek (Eds.), Learning and its disorders. Vol. 1, the Langley Porter Child Psychiatry Series. Palo Alto, Calif.: Science and Behavior Books, 1965.

5. LOWREY, L. G. Trends in therapy, evolution, status, and trends. Amer. J. Orthopsychiat. 9:669-706, 1939.

6. ROGERS, C. The clinical treatment of the problem child. New York: Houghton Mifflin, 1939.

7. SZUREK, S. A. Notes on the genesis of psychopathic personality trends. Psychiatry, 5:1-6, 1942. (See page 3 of this volume.)

8. SZUREK, S. A., JOHNSON, A. M., & FALSTEIN, E. I. Collaborative psychiatric therapy of parent-child problems. Amer. J. Orthopsychiat., 12:511-516, 1942. Reprinted in S. A. Szurek & I. N. Berlin (Eds.), Training in therapeutic work with children. Vol. 2, the Langley Porter Child Psychiatry Series. Palo Alto, Calif.: Science and Behavior Books, 1967.

9. TANNEBAUM, F. Crime and the community. New York: Ginn and Co., 1938.

THE CONTROL OF ACTING-OUT
IN THE PSYCHOTHERAPY OF DELINQUENTS*

Maurice Kaplan, John F. Ryan, Edward Nathan,
and Marion Bairos

The problem of delinquency is a perennial concern in our
society and we are never permitted to ignore it. Early in the
century this concern led to the development of the child guidance
movement; hopes were high that the application of newly developed
psychodynamic concepts would prove to be the answer to the problem. Unfortunately, these hopes were not borne out.

The problem is too great to be solved by psychotherapy alone.
The viewpoints regarding etiology are many, and the methods
suggested and attempted for prophylaxis, as well as correction,
are equally varied. By its very nature psychotherapy can have
only limited application and is only one approach to the problem
of delinquency. The solution of this problem will require the
application of techniques based upon sociological, cultural, medical, and economic, as well as psychological, premises. Nevertheless, we believe that the clear elucidation of psychological principles derived from psychotherapeutic work with delinquents can
find application in approaches other than the strictly psychotherapeutic.

When psychotherapy for the delinquent was first proposed, it
was felt that the method and course of treatment would not differ
materially from that with neurotics. This hope was soon frustrated. The methods developed in work with the more typical neurotic
have not proven applicable to the delinquent. Most clinics have had
disappointing experience with psychotherapy of delinquents. Of the
number who come on a voluntary basis, relatively few—delinquents
or families—continue in treatment long enough for the desired
character changes to take place.

---

*Reprinted with permission from American Journal of Psychiatry,
113:1108-14, 1957.

Initially, we want to make clear that we are not using the term "delinquent" in a diagnostic sense. We agree with those who object to its diagnostic use, believing that it is mainly a descriptive, social and legal term. We use it here because we are not now concerned with any precise psychopathological differentiation between the various personality disorders in which delinquent behavior may occur, but rather with that general category of cases where delinquent behavior is a persistent and prominent symptom, regardless of the specific psychopathological picture intensive study may later reveal. We are mainly interested with the one trait common to all such disorders.

Nor are we concerned with the question of whether certain forms of delinquent behavior are primarily sociologically determined as opposed to such behavior produced by internal conflict. In our opinion, an attempt at this kind of distinction has little merit. Whatever factors we may consider as etiologically important—whether constitutional, social, economic, or cultural—their influence is finally upon the mental life of the individual, his psychological structure and function. The delinquent act is determined by a psychological state, and we must therefore discuss it in psychological terms. We must strive to make a psychodynamic formulation.

DYNAMICS OF THE DELINQUENT

We would like to review briefly some general dynamic characteristics, more or less true of patients in whom delinquent behavior is a prominent symptom. The most striking is that the delinquent does not appear to suffer in the same way and in the same circumstances as does the neurotic. The suffering of the delinquent is usually a result of external circumstances and continues only so long as those circumstances are present. He suffers largely from his environment, the neurotic from sources within himself. Another way of saying this is that the delinquent does not seem to have the capacity for building up and storing anxiety—at least not to the point where it is experienced as discomfort, localized internally, and consciously felt as coming from within. It tends to be discharged through action before or immediately after the threshold of discomfort is reached. Since consciously felt anxiety is the prime motivating force in psychotherapy, it is his inability to contain and experience anxiety that makes work with the delinquent so difficult to initiate and so dubious prognostically.

In addition, once therapy is begun, the capacity for and the quality of the transference differentiate between the delinquent and the neurotic. To clarify this point requires some further distinction between these two large categories of disturbance. Basically, the neurotic has a passive-receptive attitude. Whatever fixations are present at other stages of psychosexual development, problems of orality are ever present and ultimately manifest themselves. Though he feels ashamed of it, struggles against it, disguises it in a multiplicity of defense mechanisms, the neurotic deeply longs for a dependent, orally receptive relationship. He resents the need, but he has not given it up entirely. Early in therapy this tends toward the development of a strong transference with a unique ambivalent tone.

The delinquent, too, has deep, unsatisfied oral longings; but in his case they have followed a different development. He has more definitely turned against them and vigorously denies them. In addition, differences are manifest in the nature of his relationship to the object. His separation and withdrawal from the object is greater, amounting to almost complete rejection. He has defiantly given up hope of freely receiving; in fact, this would be too danger-ous. He has angrily turned against the object but defensively he regards the object as having turned against him—the object is not only depriving and rejecting, but an enemy to be guarded against. The delinquent, however, has not given up hope of obtaining some-thing from the object, but he does not expect it to be freely given. In fact, a passive role is too dangerous and is rigorously avoided. Therefore, he schemes to take what he wants by force or trickery, and the object thus becomes a victim, "a sucker," that he will ex-ploit. In effect, the delinquent says, "I'll get mine by hook or by crook," hoping to satisfy his wishes and at the same time wreak vengeance on the object. His guilt is assuaged in advance by the basic feeling of the fantasied wrong. His attitude is, "I'm taking my chances and risking my neck."

The problem of orality in these two large categories can perhaps be summarized as follows: The neurotic distrusts and deeply hopes he will be proven wrong; the delinquent distrusts and is afraid he will be proven wrong. On the deepest level, as in all that is human, the delinquent and neurotic are not too different. The need to trust is there, no matter how vestigial. If this were not so, there would be little point in talking about the psychotherapy of delinquents.

Another important difference is the relative capacity to divide the ego into an experiencing part and an observing part. Fenichel refers to it as the detachment of the reasonable ego from the de-fensive ego. In everyday language we would call it the capacity for ordered and rational introspection. This capacity the neurotic typically possesses to a high degree, often even before therapy, though it is then usually of a ruminative and anxiety-ridden kind. The neurotic, in a sense, is tuned in on his inner experiences, and this characteristic can be utilized in therapy to develop a discriminating self-observation and self-awareness. In the delinquent, this quality is vestigial, if present at all; the delinquent is more likely tuned in on the object, and his often remarkably keen intuitive insights regarding the other person are more accessible to his awareness.

Closely related to this quality is the way projection manifests itself in the delinquent. In contrast to the neurotic and psychotic, it is not the impulse which is projected, that is readily accepted as his own, but rather the genesis of the impulse and the circumstances of its expression. The misdeed is blamed on circumstances, bad companions, temptation, provocation by the victim, or similar factors. This is extremely difficult to deal with in therapy, since there is nearly always an element of truth in the projection, which stems from the primary traumatic situation and is confirmed by the subsequent retaliatory and vengeful attitudes he has encountered.

The difference between the neurotic and the delinquent is related not only to superego development—its exaggerated, harsh quality in the neurotic and its stunted or lacunar maldevelopment in the delinquent. There are similar differences in ego development, in the nature of the perception of external reality, in the quality of memory, and in the capacity to integrate new experiences. Both ego and superego development are determined to a great extent by the type and quality of the identifications which have taken place, and, further, by the kind of self-image or ego identity which has developed.

ANXIETY AND ACTING-OUT

As we emphasized earlier, the psychopathological characteristic of the delinquent that is of the main concern to us in the development of our thesis is his inability to endure anxiety and his tendency to impulsively discharge it in action. The tendency of the delinquent to act out his conflicts is the chief obstacle to psychotherapy. We believe it is axiomatic that acting-out and psychotherapy are antithetical to and bear an inverse relationship to each other. The problem then becomes to establish conditions, short of incarceration, which will reduce the possibility of acting-out. In a sense, our psychodynamic considerations parallel the more simply stated premises of society: in the guise of our psychiatric jargon we are restating commonly known truisms. When we say that an important characteristic of the delinquent is his tendency to act out, we are simply saying that the delinquent has a tendency to commit delinquent acts. Of course, this is an oversimplification, and in a psychopathological sense we intend much more by the term "acting-out."

Nevertheless, it is the age-old common sense recognition of this problem that has operated in the development of our penal system, (which does not deny the retaliatory and vengeful features that were and still are associated with our methods of dealing with antisocial behavior). It is also true, however, that, as society increasingly masters these anxiously retaliatory and vengeful tendencies, its attitudes toward the management of crime and criminals more closely approximate the viewpoints of psychiatry. Though society as a whole is still a long way from viewing delinquency, much less crime, from the standpoint of health and disease, the punitive, vengeful attitudes, which are now dominant features in the organization and operation of our penal system, in the future may be seen as the destructive, irrational products of our own anxieties. In that Utopian era, such tendencies will, hopefully, be recognized and dealt with much as dynamic psychiatrists now deal with countertransference in therapeutic work.

Let us examine the problem of the treatment of delinquents in terms of ego function, just as we do in the case of other, less antisocial mental illnesses. The need for external controls would be determined by a clinical estimate of the individual's capacity to control his impulses toward antisocial behavior. Probation, the circumstance under which most delinquents come to us, may be regarded as a method of stimulating greater ego control in lieu of the application of external controls by incarceration. The coercion effected through imprisonment, as well as through parole or probation, is directed at the antisocial acting-out impulses of the individual. Since the delinquent's ego has not sufficiently integrated his antisocial tendencies, these measures, though crude, must be substituted by society for his own inadequately functioning ego. It is our contention that when such controls are instituted and carried out on a rational basis, with careful attention to the correction and exclusion of retaliatory tendencies in all concerned, they need not necessarily interfere with psychotherapy. It is important to acknowledge that such controls, contrary to what is too often told the delinquent, are not primarily for his own good, but are first of all for the protection of society. If any other reason is presented, it can only be regarded by the delinquent as not quite genuine. Providing they are freed of overtones of retaliation, the controls are not in opposition to the true interests of the delinquent. They do not in themselves represent a hostile infringement of his rights, nor are they an unjustified interference with the satisfaction of his usual needs. Ideally, the delinquent is provided with a choice: to modify his actions (not his feelings) in accordance with the requirements of society, or to lose a large measure of his self-determination.

COMPULSORY PSYCHOTHERAPY

At our clinic, we encourage the inclusion of compulsory psychotherapy as one of the conditions of probation. We do not look upon
it as a substitute for probation, nor the relationship with the psychotherapist as a substitute for that with the probation officer. We
definitely encourage the probation officer to continue the same
routine as would obtain without psychotherapy. We do not believe
his function is one that need interfere in any way with the psychotherapeutic program. Furthermore, we feel that close collaboration between the probation officer and the clinic team is an
essential feature of the total program.

As previously indicated, our hypothesis is that the more that
acting-out by the delinquent can be prevented, the less the anxiety
that can be discharged in that way. Concomitant psychotherapy
thus provides an alternative avenue for the discharge of anxiety,
though not one of which the delinquent can immediately and readily
make full use. The easy route of acting-out is not given up without
a struggle. Naturally, the qualifications of the therapist are important factors at this point, and most important is the quality of the
collaboration between the therapist and probation officer. Lack of
communication and unresolved differences between them tend to
create a gap through which the delinquent may escape into some
form of acting-out.

The problem in the outpatient treatment of the delinquent is to
control the acting-out by purely psychological means. This is
partly met by the conditions of probation which have been clearly
defined to him. It further calls for the delinquent and his parents
to be regularly confronted with the reality situation. This entails
the clarification of all courses of action from which he may choose
with the probable and possible consequences of each one openly and
thoroughly discussed. It means the alternate choices and their
consequences are spelled out at appropriate times with neither
retaliatory nor guilty overtones, but simply as a definition of his
reality. The position of the therapist is, as always, to oppose the
self-destructive impulses of the patient and unequivocally to nurture
the constructive, genuinely ego-syntonic tendencies.

In order to be effective in controlling the acting-out tendencies
of the delinquent, it is not enough to have a good understanding of
his psychopathology. That, of course, is important; we do not
minimize it. But, in addition, in order to deal adequately with his
tendency to act-out, we must observe and understand how the delinquent and the significant people around him interact with one
another. (Here, when we speak of the delinquent, we are referring
to the constellation of child and parent or parents—the "delinquent

constellation.") The significant people, other than the parents, include therapists, probation officers, teachers, and others with whom the delinquent relates, even if only briefly and temporarily. We are interested in the nature of the transactions between the delinquent constellation and each of the others which may, in some way, encourage or discourage the tendency to act out. We are concerned about the transactions between all those persons involved with the delinquent constellation which may serve a similar purpose. These transactions frequently center around a single issue which may seem critical at the time, and upon the resolution of this issue, directly or indirectly, frequently hinges the fate of the psychotherapeutic work, its continuation or disruption.

For example, the question, usually initiated by the delinquent constellation, may be whether the boy might join the armed services, or whether he should move to another city where an employer has been found who has taken a special interest in him. Or, it may be whether he should continue in school or take a job. These issues are seemingly innocent and temptingly valid steps in themselves, and certainly are consciously felt that way by all involved. Yet, they often carry within them the seed of the delinquent's resistance. In addition to other meanings, we have come to regard such issues as often being the verbal signal of the acting-out tendency. At this point the attitudes and activities, both conscious and unconscious, of all those involved with the delinquent become critically important. These individuals can contribute in an important way to the active expression or the early prevention of the acting-out.

THE IMPORTANCE OF COLLABORATION

It is here that collaboration, carried on through conferences, becomes extremely important: its nature can determine the fate of the work with the delinquent constellation. A clear understanding of the interpersonal dynamics involving all the people concerned is as important as an understanding of the intrapsychic dynamics of the delinquent. This is particularly important for the therapist whose attention must at all times include both the delinquent and the delinquent constellation. He must be alert, not only to what the delinquent is signalling during his therapy hour, but also to what is being communicated in the interaction between all the people involved. All of these activities finally bear upon the psychotherapeutic work. Beyond the basic nature of the defense structure of the delinquent, it is the relationships between all those who are significantly involved with him that influence the fluid balance of impulse and defense and, therefore, the strength of the acting-out tendency. We know that in certain phases of psychotherapy with any patient, inner forces are mobilized which, if not given sufficient verbal expression, may lead to disruption of therapy or other types of acting-out. An example of this is the anxiety produced by increasingly dependent feelings. When this occurs in the delinquent, and if a seemingly reasonable exit is coincidentally offered, it is likely that the delinquent will take the exit and thus break off therapy. It is our feeling that more attention to the dynamic understanding of what we can call the collaborative aspects of the treatment of the delinquent, and an attempt to improve the collaboration, may lead to improved results.

By means of brief excerpts from several cases, we shall illustrate some of the situations which can occur in collaborative work and which seem to have a bearing on the acting-out tendency of the delinquent.

Following repeated delinquent acts, a sixteen-year-old boy was offered by the court the choice of probation and outpatient treatment as an alternative to placement in a custodial institution. Although choosing probation and complying with the directive to obtain psychotherapeutic help, his mother openly expressed her skepticism regarding its value. In her sessions at the clinic she minced no words in expressing her objections to the coercion and attacked the therapists and court workers with sarcasm. Her son maintained a similar attitude and was arrogant and defiant. In various ways he repeatedly attempted to provoke the therapist. After two months of therapy, the mother wrote the probation officer, objecting to therapy and suggesting that the boy be allowed to see a priest instead. She argued that a priest would not attribute all their problems to sex, as we would. The probation officer was uncertain and hesitated to insist that the family comply with this requirement of probation, saying, "You can't force it down their throats." He further suggested that, since the boy had not been involved in any delinquencies for several months, he had perhaps had enough treatment. At a conference called to redefine the respective roles of the clinic and the court, the court's representatives expressed surprise that we were willing to undertake treatment of patients under conditions of coercion. They decided, however, to meet the mother's maneuver by offering her the alternative of continued treatment or another court hearing to reconsider the situation.

When met with calm firmness, despite her storming and arguing, she and her son continued in therapy. This is not meant to imply that the problem was settled finally, and that treatment then proceeded to a successful conclusion. In this particular case, our efforts were ultimately not successful, for the boy by repeated, flagrant delinquencies finally forced the authorities to place him in an institution. We cite this case merely as an example of a rather common situation that can lead to disruption of treatment. It illustrates how the delinquent consciously or unconsciously tests for differences between the various agencies with whom he is involved and proceeds to exploit them.

At one point, the patient and his mother informed their therapists that the boy had planned a visit with his godfather in another town. What they had not revealed, and about which the therapists did not inquire, was that they had not consulted the probation officer whose province it was to grant permission to leave the city. (This kind of communication, when it does catch the attention of the therapist, offers a useful opportunity for confronting the patients with their defiant attitudes, both for a clarification of their relationship with their therapists and with the court, and for much more that is pertinent to treatment.) It is interesting that, following this, the mother again approached the probation officer with the proposal that they be allowed to discontinue treatment, and the boy be allowed to remain in the other town where, in lieu of his therapist, he could "talk" with his godfather, with whom he presumably had a good relationship. This proposal was dealt with in an essentially similar way to the preceding one, but much more quickly and with much smoother collaboration.

These illustrations indicate how the delinquent may announce an intended action which seems to be of no particular significance, but on closer examination may have an important bearing on tendencies which threaten to erupt into action. This kind of communication is also related to the subtle ways in which the delinquent may involve his therapist as a passive accomplice in a germinating delinquency. A better way of stating this, perhaps, is that the delinquent signals the presence of a delinquent impulse. The various ways in which the delinquent's communication can be understood are all probably in some way correct and no doubt represent the multiple determinants of the communication. These include the conflicting forces struggling within him, ranging from the wish for help in controlling his impulses to the defiant challenge to stop him—and as in all conflict the two extremes are strongly interlocked.

The final delinquencies which led to this boy's imprisonment followed almost immediately an independent decision by the probation officer to shorten the period of probation so that the boy could join the Navy. It is interesting that one of his final acts was to send to a neighbor a clumsy extortion note (which practically pointed to him), in which he claimed $100 was due him "for a month of protection." Our own question would be: was the boy using this note to say that he was not yet ready for the relative independence of life in the Navy?

Another episode in this case illustrated dramatically how the

parent is often involved in the child's delinquency, both actually as
well as psychologically. One day the boy came home with a relatively new Buick and offered his mother a ride, saying he had
borrowed the car from a friend. Though vaguely uneasy about his
story and aware that he did not possess a driver's license, she
accompanied him. That same evening he was arrested for the theft
of the car. This vignette is of the same order as another: the
mother of a nursery school child, when called to school and informed that her son had bitten another child, turned helplessly to
him and chided, "Why did you bite so hard?"

It is in instances such as these that the parent's own poorly
integrated aggressive-rebellious impulses become apparent, and
are often expressed at critical moments in uncertain, somewhat
confused responses. It's as if the child were asking, "How do you
feel about my reactions?" And the parent responds with, "I don't
know—part of me secretly applauds you."

We might point out that the therapist, too, is confronted by the
same problem—we refer to his own aggressive-rebellious tendencies—and the degree to which he has already solved it for himself
will determine to a great extent his inner unity and, therefore, the
clarity with which he deals with the delinquent and his family. In
discussing another patient, who at the point of a knife had demanded
money from two younger children, a therapist at one time referred
to the act as the "so-called armed robbery," and again as "just a
silly act." In a later discussion of this case, the therapist raised
the question of to whose side, court's or patient's, a therapist had
to be on. This, of course, is a false issue—since it implies the
premise that the needs of the individual are necessarily opposed to
the needs of society, and that the two cannot be adjusted to the
benefit of both. The attitude revealed bears a close similarity to
that shown by the parents in the earlier examples cited. In such
instances, it seems that the necessary empathy for all the feelings
of the patient, including his aggressive, defiant and rebellious ones,
is not sufficiently discriminated from one's own residual guilt,
overidentification, or other countertransference manifestations. It
is the latter that interferes with a relatively realistic evaluation of
the delinquent's acting-out. To paraphase Voltaire, the therapist
of the delinquent needs to be able to say: "I strongly disagree with
the expression of your aggressive impulses in action, but will
defend your right to feel them."

Another adolescent boy, in struggling with dependent transference
feelings, threatened to quit therapy and join the Merchant Marine.
Without prior consultation with us, the probation officer was induced
to give him written permission to do so. That this request was an
expression of the transference was suggested when the patient de-

manded of his therapist similar written permission, even though
such permission was unnecessary. The therapist first responded
by expressing his disagreement with the move. In further exploration, he confirmed his own suspicion that the patient knew that his
permission was not needed officially. A conference was held with
the probation officer who at first defended his move and expressed
the idea that the Merchant Marine might "make a man of him." He
recalled another delinquent with whom he had worked, who was now
a captain in the Merchant Marine. But, when all the pertinent material had been reviewed, he agreed that he had perhaps acceded too
quickly to the boy's demand.

Similar examples of the types of transaction that commonly occur
between the delinquent and all those involved with him could be mul-
tiplied. The situations are exceedingly varied, though resembling
each other in essential features. The interplay between the acting-
out tendency and the growing strength of the transference is well
illustrated in the case of the boy who threatened to join the Merchant
Marine. His positive feelings toward his therapist were rather obvious, and that his struggles were increasingly against them was often
equally clear. At one time he absentmindedly came to the clinic on
a holiday, when the clinic was closed, and then failed to keep the
alternate appointment that had been arranged for him. In arguing
for the Merchant Marine, he protested, "I only see you one hour a
week, and even if I saw you all day every day, I would still want to
join up. School doesn't want me, and I don't want to come here until
I'm twenty-five." In demanding the therapist's written permission
and acknowledging that it wasn't officially necessary, he insisted
that the therapist was still "a bottleneck." During one period in
therapy he was repeatedly seen waiting in front of the closed clinic
at about 8:00 A.M. for an 8:30 appointment. Later, he told his
mother that he would never come early again: "They might get the
idea that I like it." Though this case, too, was no shining success,
similar evidence in other cases as well leads us to suspect that the
compulsory treatment of delinquents can be more successful than
commonly supposed.

In the treatment of delinquents on an outpatient basis, we are
suggesting the deliberate extension of the team concept beyond the
walls of the clinic to include the probation officer, the school, and
the pertinent social agencies. That this presents difficulties, that
the work is at times discouraging, that it complicates the clearly
defined and pleasant privacy of the one-to-one relationship in the
interview room, are no doubt true. But, since the treatment of
delinquents has heretofore never been particularly encouraging,
every well-considered idea is worthy of an adequate clinical trial.

SUGGESTED ADDITIONAL READINGS

1. CURRAN, F. J.A.M.A., 157:108, 1955.
2. FENICHEL, O. Psychoanal. Quart., 1947.
3. FREUD, A. The ego and the mechanisms of defense. London: Hogarth Press, 1937.
4. FURMAN, S. S. (Ed.), Reaching the unreached. New York: New York City Youth Board, 1952.
5. JOHNSON, A. M., & SZUREK, S. A. Psychoanal. Quart., 21:323, 1952.
6. STANTON, H., & SCHWARTZ, M. H. Psychiatry, 12:13, 1949.
7. SZUREK, S. A. Emotional factors in the use of authority. In Public health is people. New York: Commonwealth Fund, 1950. (See page 48 of this volume.)
8. WHITAKER, C. Psychiatry, 9:239, 1946

PSYCHOLOGICAL ASPECTS OF
GLUE-SNIFFING BY JUVENILES*

John Langdell

Glue-sniffing behavior is the deliberate inhalation of the volatile solvents of plastic cement for an intoxicating effect. This practice has become widespread, particularly among boys between seven and sixteen years of ages. The usual volatile solvents in quick-drying glues are toluene and acetone, which have effects on the central nervous system similar to alcohol, ether, or chloroform. Glues containing toluene have been most popular because acetone has a more disagreeable odor. The fumes of glue are inhaled from a handkerchief or bag until a drunken state or unconsciousness results. Boys under the influence of glue have done such things as jumping off a building in an attempt to fly, assuming a fighting stance in front of an oncoming freight train, single-handedly attacking four marines, and stealing cars for joy riding (27). A stuporous state is a more frequent result. Persistent glue-sniffers may be recognized by their bloodshot eyes, running noses, excessive salivation, and foul-smelling breath with an odor of glue.

The glue-sniffing behavior of modern juveniles is one of the latest manifestations of mankind's age-old search for chemical agents to provide peace of mind, relief from tension, and escape from unpleasant reality. Since prehistoric times people on every continent have been using drugs in strange and varied ways in efforts to attain instant happiness. The Odyssey tells of the lotus-eaters who became "forgetful of their homeward way," and of Helen, who cast a drug into the wine "to lull all pain and anger and bring forgetfulness of every sorrow." Herodotus wrote in his history 2,400 years ago of the Scythians who, to cause drunkenness, sat around a fire sniffing the smoke of hashish plants which they threw on the fire. After sniffing the smoke, they would jump up and begin to dance and sing. Modern chemical technology has made available

---

*Unpublished 1968.

many new substances for such experimentation, while the rapidity of modern communication and transportation has insured immediate spread of the latest fads of drug usage. Although abuses of such agents as alcohol, hashish, opium, tobacco, peyote, tea, and coffee are prehistoric, there has been no period in history when drug usage has been so prevalent as in the current burst of experimentation by adolescents and young adults (25).

In the few years since 1960, when glue-sniffing was first described in the American medical literature (2)—sniffing practices were first reported in Sweden several years earlier (3)—it has become a widespread problem, and public alarm has resulted in legislation to regulate it. In some aspects glue-sniffing is actually a more serious problem than the use of illegal narcotics. The most alarming aspect is its prevalence among children at a younger age level than are ordinarily exposed to opiates, marijuana, barbiturates, alcohol, hallucinogenic agents, and other widely used drugs. The fact that the material used—model airplane type plastic glue—is so readily available to young children makes its control most difficult.

Actual physical addiction with withdrawal symptoms has been reported from glue-sniffing (19) as well as at least nine deaths (27). Glue-sniffing is said to be a more frequent step toward narcotic usage than is marijuana, which has been illegal in the U. S. only since 1937 and is reported to be neither an addictive drug itself nor a serious channel to other addictions (10). It is a social paradox that about six thousand persons are at present in California prisons on marijuana charges, although the substance is reportedly nonaddicting and is a less serious threat to life and health than is glue, or the more socially acceptable alcohol and tobacco. Since glue-sniffing has caused death, brain injury, and kidney damage, it appears to be more of a threat to physical health than are narcotics, regarding which it has been recently written: "There is no evidence that the prolonged use of any opiate in and of itself causes any physical pathology" (10). However, physical pathology of brain, kidney, lung, and blood-forming organs has been reported from glue-sniffing and inhalation of toluene, the usual solvent in glue (13, 17, 22,24,27). There has been an absence of hematological or urinary pathology in the case reports of some workers (1,12).

The sale of glue has been regulated by such laws as California Assembly Bill No. 349, passed on June 12, 1965, which makes it illegal to sell glue or cement containing toluene or any substance with toxic qualities similar to toluene to any person who is less than eighteen years of age unless "the glue or cement is sold, delivered, or given away simultaneously with or as part of a kit used for the construction of model airplanes, model boats, model automobiles, model trains, or other similar models." A number of cities, counties, and states have enacted laws against glue-sniffing (27).

Glue-sniffing behavior is similar to some other fads popular in the past. In the period following World War I, gasoline-sniffing was a widespread problem (4,7,8,9,16,21,23). Nutmeg has occasionally been ingested for the purpose of intoxication, only five grams having a profound effect on the individual (5,11,14,23, 26,28,29). A one-time craze among college students and faculty for the sniffing of chloroform, ether, or nitrous oxide led to the practical application of such agents in surgical anesthesia. For a modern variation, compressed nitrous oxide gas that is sold to restaurants to produce whipped cream has been used to provide a "bag full of laughs" at parties (6). Other substances that are sniffed for intoxicating effects include fingernail polish, lighter fluid, and felt-pen ink.

The juvenile practice of glue-sniffing parallels the current widespread usage of psychoactive agents by members of an older age group. The use of such substances as LSD, mescaline, peyote, morning glory seeds and marijuana has been popularized by a "consciousness-expanding" cult, which may be in the process of becoming an organized religion. Historically, such substances have been widely used in religious rituals: Polynesian women chewed kava roots to prepare a ceremonial beverage for their men; certain Eskimos drank one another's urine so none of the effects of an ingested psychotoxic substance would be wasted; North American Indian tribes used peyote, Jimson weed, and tobacco for religious purposes, while Mexicans ingested sacred mushrooms. Alcoholic beverages have been involved in ancient Greek and modern Christian religious ceremonies, although their most frequent and widespread use is for purely pleasurable effects. "Virtually every nonliterate society investigated by anthropologists has utilized drugs in one form or another, largely for their hedonistic effects (20)."

The glue-sniffing fad spread rapidly throughout the United States between 1960 and 1962, when two national news magazines had feature articles on the subject. An editorial in the British Medical Journal discussed the fad and noted there were no cases reported in England. However, a few months later the first English case was reported—the man had learned about glue-sniffing from an American magazine (19).

CASE REPORTS

The author first became aware of the clinical problem of glue-sniffing in 1960, early in the development of the fad, in the course

of psychotherapeutic work with a boy who was confined in a juvenile institution following arrest for numerous episodes of breaking
and entering.

This sixteen-year-old boy had repeatedly broken into vacant sum-
mer homes to drink up the liquor supply while watching television.
In some of the homes he caused property damage by throwing bot-
tles and other objects. He consistently denied the involvement of
anyone else in the thefts, although he had been apprehended as a
consequence of supplying stolen beer to other boys. He explained
that his solitary activity was a quiet relief from his home situation
where he felt displaced by a young sibling. He experienced considerable strain in his relationship with his parents, particularly with
his father, a college professor who had become so disappointed at
his son's unsatisfactory school performance that he had lost all interest in the boy and felt no warmth toward him. Both parents had
been distressed for years at his poor academic performance in
spite of his superior intelligence. Several years previously the
parents had consulted the author about their son's underachieve-
ment in school. There had been some improvement during a period of concomitant interviews with the boy and both parents; but the
treatment program, financially limited to brief and infrequent interviews, was interrupted when the birth of a baby brought further
financial limitations. When the boy was arrested, his parents requested additional therapy and made arrangements to bring the boy
to the office from the juvenile home in which he was confined. A
probation officer provided conjoint family therapy interviews and
worked collaboratively with the author.

The boy immediately resumed his previous therapeutic relationship and spoke freely. In one of the early sessions he told of being
very busy working with other boys in the institution making model
airplanes. With a sardonic smile he described in detail how he and
the other boys kept staff members busy supplying them with more
glue. He described with some glee how he enjoyed getting drunk
by sniffing the glue, knowing he was making suckers out of the staff
members who were encouraging the boys' model-making hobby.
When he expressed some concern that he felt a little sick after
sniffing glue, the therapist expressed his own concern that the
poisonous solvents in the glue might damage his brain, liver, or
other organs. The boy later reported he had told the other boys
his doctor had advised him not to sniff glue, and they had moved
on to other activities. He did not participate in further glue-
sniffing, but he did continue to have occasional alcoholic sprees
after his release. He went to work during his probation period
to earn money to make financial restitution for some of the

damage he had done. Treatment was interrupted by his entry into military service.

Glue-sniffing involved only a transitory incident in this boy's general pattern of neurotic learning disorder and delinquent acting-out behavior. That glue-sniffing behavior per se may be a severe problem is illustrated in the following case summary of a younger boy's behavior: A school principal telephoned late on a Friday night and revealed his concern about his eleven-year-old son, who had been sniffing glue for more than a year. Each time when caught the boy had faithfully promised to stop. Now after a year of such behavior the father realized his boy could not stop without professional help: he had just discovered the boy lying unconscious on the living-room floor with a glue-soaked paper bag in his hand.

He described the boy as very unhappy and lonely. Without friends of his own, he had tagged after his older brother and had gotten involved in glue-sniffing with his brother and his friends. He had continued to sniff glue alone after all the other boys had lost interest in such behavior. Most of the time he was listless or irritable, and his school performance had dropped alarmingly. The father accepted an appointment to come to the office the next day with his wife and son, and expressed relief at finally having help with this problem which had worried him for so long. Early the next morning he telephoned to cancel the appointment, explaining that his son had promised never to sniff glue again if he could just be excused from seeing a psychiatrist. The father seemed sure the problem was solved. There was no further contact, but it seems unlikely that they lived happily ever after.

Unlike most cases reported, both these boys were of middle-class backgrounds, and as it happens both were sons of educators. Both were of white ancestry (glue-sniffing is rarely reported among Negroes). Boys of teen and preteen age are most frequently involved in glue-sniffing, although girls are occasionally talked into it by boys.

The following case is reported in more detail because of the wealth of clinical information available from long-term therapy of the boy and his parents and from collaborative work with school and probation departments. Previously published reports of psychological factors in glue-sniffing are based on information obtained in only a few interviews. No prior reports of psychotherapeutic work with glue-sniffers have been found, although authors do recommed psychotherapy or at least psychological study for glue-sniffers (1,12,18).

Glue-sniffing behavior by the following child was so serious that it led to his incarceration. Psychotherapeutic work with the boy and his parents, as well as collaborative work with the boy's probation officer, enabled the elimination of glue-sniffing behavior and other serious delinquencies. The general method was a form of compulsory psychotherapy with close collaboration between probation officer and therapist as described in Chapter 8 of this volume.

This sixteen-year-old, white, American, Catholic schoolboy was brought to the clinic by his parents after he was suspended from school for the fourteenth time. The school had made psychiatric care a prerequisite for his return to school. (The current expulsion followed his attacking another boy in the schoolyard and knocking him unconscious.) Since his first day in kindergarten, when he was dragged screaming to school, he had a long history of poor school adjustment with antisocial and destructive behavior. At the age of nine years he had his first trouble with the law, being arrested for stealing checks from the mail. This happened about the time his parents were divorced. Repeated offenses included truancy, breaking school windows, using foul language, refusing to participate in physical education, and aggressive behavior toward Negro students. He had attended a total of twelve different schools and had been committed to a state hospital as a result of his disturbed behavior. Soon after the latest suspension from school he was arrested for beating a store clerk who refused to sell him cigarettes.

The boy lived with his mother, who was employed full time as a clerk, and occasionally saw his father, who provided no financial support. The father, who was working as a parking-lot attendant, formerly had been a school principal until alcoholism led him three times into a state hospital. A sister three years older was married and lived outside the home. The patient was the middle of three brothers, one a year older and the other two years younger than he. The other children had behavior problems, but none as severe as his. His paternal grandfather was a successful businessman and an influential member of the community. Glue-sniffing behavior, which had started six months previously, became uncontrolled after the sudden and unexpected death of the grandfather.

It was not known at the time of the initial diagnostic evaluation that the boy was engaged in glue-sniffing. This diagnostic evaluation included a physical examination, a neurological examination, x-rays, electroencephalograms, and laboratory study. The findings were normal with the exception of albumin in the urine on two occasions and an abnormal electroencephalogram. The electroencephalogram showed paroxysmal dysrhythmia indicating organic brain disorder. When it became known that the boy had been sniffing glue, the tests were repeated. He had a normal urine and normal Addis count after he stopped glue-sniffing, but the electro-encephalogram remained abnormal a year later.

In the course of the psychiatric study it was arranged for the boy and parents to begin psychotherapeutic interviews as soon as treatment time would become available. Ironically, the boy was remanded to a juvenile institution the day before his first sched-uled interview. After sniffing glue, he had returned home where he threatened his brother and then began sniffing chloroform. He became wilder, more threatening, and uncontrollable in his behav-ior, and drove his fist through a window. After he began making suicidal threats, his mother finally called the police. He was sent to a state institution as beyond parental control, and while he was still confined, therapeutic work was started with his parents. The mother kept her appointments regularly, but the father failed to keep over half of his first seventeen scheduled interviews and then dropped out of treatment to return to a state hospital on an alco-holic commitment.

When the boy returned from the institution, he was late for his appointments. When he failed an appointment with his therapist and also with his probation officer, the officer had him picked up by the police and held for several days. This firm stand by the probation officer clearly established that treatment really was a condition of his probation, and the boy settled down to quite regular use of his weekly therapeutic hours over the next two years. Al-though he had a series of six different probation officers, he had the same therapist, and continued collaboration and communication was maintained between the therapist and each probation officer. With this external control the boy's serious delinquency was con-tained. At the time of this writing the boy has made a transition to a new therapist, and the probation officer is considering termi-nating the probation. The boy has become so engaged in therapy that it seems likely he will continue without compulsion. The mother has continued her psychotherapeutic interviews over the two-year period as well.

Glue-sniffing behavior still occurred at the beginning of treat-ment but was gradually discontinued and stopped completely in the first year of psychotherapy. In talking of his sniffing, the boy said it made him forget any worries about the present or future. When he sniffed glue, he was able to forget everything that bothered him and he insisted adamantly that glue-sniffing was nothing like drinking. He had tried drinking but did not like it at all, and drunks disgusted him: he could not stand his drunken father. He said, "A drunk is no man at all." He mentioned that he began sniffing glue more fre-quently after his grandfather died and wondered why that was so.

Therapeutic work with the parents and collaborative work with

112

probation officers was an important aspect of treatment. The probation officer's firm stand early in treatment limited acting-out and forced the boy to attend interviews long enough to develop self-motivation after he had experienced some personal benefit. It would probably have been impossible to engage the boy in treatment without this external pressure.

Children who become habituated to glue-sniffing are frequently involved in forms of juvenile asocial behavior (12), exhibit some degree of chronic depression, and relate to peers and authorities in a passive-aggressive manner (18). Their personality characteristics have been compared to alcoholics and drug addicts, who are not very amenable to psychotherapeutic treatment because the impulsive nature of their disorder causes them to deal with anxiety by flight, withdrawal, and narcosis. Impulsive children are particularly difficult to treat in office interviews unless some external controls are present and this difficulty may explain the lack of reports of psychotherapeutic work with them. Collaborative work with parents, teachers, probation officers, and others may be a necessary aspect of psychotherapeutic work with glue-sniffing children.

REFERENCES

1. BARMAN, M. L., SIGAL, N. B., BEEDLE, B., & LARSON, R. K. Acute and chronic effects of glue sniffing. Calif. Med., 100:19-22, 1964.

2. BREWER, W. R., PICCHIONE, A. L., & CHIN, L. Hazards of intentional inhalation of plastic cement fumes. Ariz. Med., 17:747-748, 1960.

3. CHRISTIANSSON, G., & KARISSON, B. Sniffing: Method of intoxication among children. Svensk. Lakartidn., 54:33-44, 1957.

4. CLINGER, O. W., & JOHNSON, N. A. Purposeful inhalation of gasoline vapors. Psychiat. Quart., 25:557-567, 1951.

5. DALE, H. H. Note on nutmeg poisoning. Proc. R. Soc. Med., 2:69-74, 1909.

6. DANTO, B. L. A bag full of laughs. Am. J. Psychiat., 121:612-613, 1964.

7. EASSON, W. M. Gasoline addiction in children. Pediatrics, 29:250-254, 1962.

8. EDWARDS, R. V. A case report of gasoline sniffing. Amer. J. Psychiat., 117:555-557, 1960.

9. FAUCETT, R. L., & JENSEN, R. A. Addiction to inhalation of gasoline fumes in children. J. Pediat., 41:364-368, 1952.

10. FREEDMAN, A. M., & WILSON, E. A. Childhood and adolescent addictive disorders. Pediatrics, 34:283-292, 425-430, 1964.

11. FÜHNER, H., WIRTH, W., & HECHT, G. Deaths from nutmeg poisoning. Medizinische Toxicologie, Stuttgart, 1951.

12. GLASER, H. H., & MASSENGALE, O. N. Glue-sniffing in children: Deliberate inhalation of vaporized plastic cements. J.A.M.A., 181:300-303, 1962.

13. GRABSKI, A. Toluene sniffing producing cerebellar degeneration. Amer. J. Psychiat., 118:461-462, 1961.

14. GREEN, R. C. Nutmeg poisoning. J.A.M.A., 171:1342-1344, 1959.

15. KAPLAN, M., RYAN, J. F., NATHAN, E., & BAIROS, M. The control of acting out in the psychotherapy of delinquents. Am. J. Psychiat., 113:1108-1114, 1957. (See page 93 of this volume.)

16. KARANI, V. Peripheral neuritis after addiction to petrol. Brit. Med. J., 5981:216, 1966.

17. MASSACHUSETTS DEPARTMENT OF PUBLIC HEALTH. Glue-sniffing by youngsters fought by department. New Eng. J. Med., 267:993-994, 1962.

18. MASSENGALE, O. N., GLASER, H. H., LELIEVRE, M. D., DODDS, J. B., & KLOCK, M. E. Physical and psychological factors in glue sniffing. New Eng. J. Med., 269:1340-1344, 1963.

19. MERRY, J., & ZACHARIADIS, N. Addiction to glue sniffing. Brit. Med. J., 2:1448, 1962.

20. MONTAGU, A. The long search for euphoria. Reflections, 1:62-69, 1966. Reprinted from The Drug Takers, Time-Life Books Special Report. New York: Time, Inc., 1965.

21. NITSCHE, C. J., & ROBINSON, J. F. Case of gasoline addiction. Amer. J. Orthopsychiat., 29:417-419, 1959.

22. POWARS, D. Aplastic anemia secondary to glue-sniffing. New Eng. J. Med., 273:700-702, 1965.

23. PRUITT, M. Bizarre intoxications. J.A.M.A., 171:2355, 1959.

24. SOKOL, J., & ROBINSON, J. L. Glue sniffing. West. Med., 4:192, 195, 196, 214, 1963.

25. STANTON, A. H. Drug use among adolescents. Am. J. Psychiat., 122:1282-1283, 1966.

26. TRUITT, E. B., CALLAWAY, E., BRAUDE, M. C., & KRANTZ, J. C. The pharmacology of myristicin: A contribution to the psychopharmacology of nutmeg. J. Neuropsychiat., 2:205-210, 1961.

27. VERHULST, H. L., & PAGE, L. A. Glue-sniffing. National Clearinghouse for Poison Control Centers Bulletin, Washington, D.C.: Govt. Printing Office, February-March 1962. Also Glue-Sniffing 11, July-August, 1964.

28. WALLACE, G. D. On nutmeg poisoning. In Contributions to Medical Research, pp. 351-364. Ann Arbor, Mich., 1903.

29. WEISS, G. Hallucinogenic and narcotic-like effects of powdered myristica (nutmeg). Psychiat. Quart., 34:346-356, 1960.

SUGGESTED ADDITIONAL READINGS

1. AKESSON, H. O., & WALINDER, J. Nutmeg intoxication. Lancet, No. 7398, 1:1271-1272, 1965.

2. ANDERSON, P., & KAADA, B. R. Electroencephalogram in poisoning by lacquer thinner (butyl acetate and toluene). Acta Pharmacol. et Toxicol., 9:125-130, 1953.

3. CORLISS, L. M. A review of the evidence on glue sniffing: A persistent problem. J. School Health, 35:442-449, 1965.

4. DODDS, J., & SANTOSTEFANO, S. A comparison of the cognitive functions of glue sniffers and non-sniffers. J. Pediat., 64:565-570, 1964.

5. DONATO, L. R., & FLUKE, B. J. Glue sniffing: Dangerous fad. Listen, 13 (3):11, 32, 1960.

6. HIFT, W., & PATEL, P. L. Acute acetone poisoning due to synthetic plaster cast. S. Afr. Med. J., 35:246-250, 1961.

7. JACOBZINER, H., & RAYBIN, J. W. Activities of poison control center in ethylene dichloride poisoning. Arch. Pediat., 78:490-495, 1961.

8. JACOBZINER, H., & RAYBIN, J. W. Accidental chemical poisoning: Glue sniffing. N.Y. State J. Med., 62:3294-3296, 1962; 16:2415-18, 1963.

9. LESTER, D. Danger—a new fad: Glue sniffing. This Week. January 20, 1963.

10. NYSWANDER, M. Drug addictions. In S. Arieti (Ed.) American Handbook of Psychiatry. New York: Basic Books, 1959.

11. PRESS, E. Glue sniffing. J. Pediat., 63:516-518, 1963.

12. PRESS, E., & DONE, A. K. Solvent sniffing. Pediatrics, 39:551-561, 611-622, 1967.

13. SATRAN, R., & DODSON, V. N. Toluene habituation. New Eng. J. Med., 268:719-721, 1963.

14. SOKOL, J. Glue sniffing. Listen, January-February 1964.

15. Editorial. Brit. Med. J., 5311:1043, 1962.
16. The new addicts. Newsweek, 60:42, August 13, 1962.
17. High on glue, lad turns thief. San Francisco News-Call Bulletin, March 27, 1963.
18. Fads: The new kick. Time, 79:55, February 16, 1962.

PROBLEMS BETWEEN A REFERRING SOURCE
AND A CHILD GUIDANCE CLINIC*

Maurice Kaplan

It is not the purpose of this paper to review the changing trends
in child psychiatry, but this brief resumé will be useful as an introduction to the subject of this paper. Early in the development of child
psychiatry the chief emphasis was placed upon the child. The child
had in some way disturbed adults in his environment, whether parents,
teachers, or legal authorities, by behavior which could be described
as aggressive, or withdrawn, or a combination of both. It is interesting to note that in the earliest days of child guidance work the
greatest concern was with overly aggressive or delinquent behavior,
a form of behavior which was disturbing chiefly to the adults in the
child's environment. In fact, the concern over this type of behavior,
which has always represented a serious social problem, was one of
the chief determinants in the genesis and development of child
guidance clinics. The child was the problem, and all the available
therapeutic resources represented by medicine, social service,
psychology, and the courts were mobilized to study the child, to
find the factors within him which caused the disturbing behavior,
and insofar as possible to correct them by suitable measures. The
family was studied mainly from the standpoint of its influence on
the child, and it was worked with to achieve changes in its organization which, it was felt, would beneficially influence the behavior
of the child. It was as if the family were regarded as an attribute
of the child, like his physical endowment and intelligence, rather
than the child as a unit in the family constellation. The psychiatric
resources utilized in trying to resolve a child's behavior problem
were mainly directed toward the child, utilizing with modifications
the one-to-one relationship traditional in adult psychotherapy. Parents were worked with through the technique of casework, but this

---

*Reprinted with permission from The Quarterly Journal of Child
Behavior, 4:80-96, 1952.

was conceived to be for the sake of the child and chiefly in order to help the parents to accept the psychotherapeutic work being done with the child.

In recent years there has been a tendency to focus equal attention on the child and his family. It is recognized that a child is referred to a clinic because of the difficulties he is causing in his environment, or because of the anxieties of people close to him; and it is still tacitly accepted that these difficulties occur because the child is emotionally disturbed. There is, however, a greater tendency to recognize the organic unity of the family, and it is suggested that the disturbance in the child is only one indication of a latent or manifest disturbance within the family. This has led to a closer study of the relationships within the family, of the mental health of each of the parents, and of the emotional difficulties they are experiencing. It is now widely felt that better results are obtainable in psychotherapeutic work with a child when at least the emotionally more significant parent is receiving treatment concomitantly. In most instances this is carried on at the same clinic and ordinarily by a therapist other than the one seeing the child. In such collaborative work difficulties are apt to occur in the course of the therapeutic work with one or more members of the family; these can be attributed, at least in part, to unresolved differences and misunderstandings between the members of the therapeutic team. The airing of such differences in conferences often serves to resolve the difficulties in therapeutic work. It has been found that regular and frequent conferences between members of the therapeutic team, with a frank discussion of any differences, are essential for the effective synchronization of their work with the family.

MEANINGS OF REFERRAL

In child guidance work a family usually comes to the clinic through referral by a social agency, a court or its adjunct services, a school, or a physician. Frequently, the agency has been helping the family in the solution of a problem for a considerable period of time prior to the referral. At some point in this work the agency comes to the conclusion that the help of a child guidance clinic may be useful. The circumstances which lead to this conclusion are variable. The agency, after a period of time, may decide that the nature of the problem which the family brought to them really requires the special approach and skills found in a clinic. Or it may feel that work of a psychotherapeutic nature for one or more members of the family is required before adequate use can be made of the service the agency has to offer. On the other hand, it may conclude that psychotherapeutic work concomitant with its own work would be helpful in resolving the family's problems. At times the agency, having reached an impasse with the family, may utilize referral as a means of obtaining consultation. There may or may not be an awareness of the impasse, and its existence may be an unrecognized factor in addition to the other more clearly appreciated reasons for referral. Whatever the reason may be, the essential point is that the referring agency and the child guidance clinic have been brought into a collaborative relationship around a given family problem.

This fact has far-reaching and important implications in the work the referring agency may continue with the family, and this is certainly true of the work the child guidance clinic has now begun with the family. The referral brings about economic changes in the dynamics of the total situation. It is certainly obvious that with an increase in the number of individuals participating in the work with a given family, the number and complexity of the dynamic factors present in the situation also increase. The relationship is now not only between the family and the referring source, but also between the family and the child guidance clinic and, through the family as well as directly, between the clinic and the referring source. One can think of this as a triangular situation involving groups somewhat analogous to the family triangular situation exemplified by the oedipus complex.

It is not the purpose of this paper to evaluate critically the desirability of this multiple approach to the handling of family problems. The historical development of our society has not only brought about the particular problems we face, but has also influenced the evolution of the institutions which deal with these problems. Naturally, an examination of the problems in relation to the associated institutions may lead to a modification of the latter to the end of greater effectiveness. My aim here is not to examine their structure, but rather to examine more closely the interrelationships of certain institutions as they now exist and operate. This may lead perhaps to greater precision in the performance of our tasks within the present institutional framework. I am raising no question, therefore, as to whether only one or several agencies should become involved in helping a single family with its problems. I am only interested in examining some of the situations which may arise in the relationship of a referring source, a family, and a clinic, and which may affect adversely or favorably the work of each in the common task of helping a particular family resolve some of its difficulties.

CLARIFYING AGENCY ROLE AND CONCERNS

The essential problem between the referring source and the clinic is what role each is to play in dealing with the family's problems. In turn the family needs to know the nature and form of help it can expect from each of the sources of help. This seems obvious and has been repeatedly described and defined in numberless publications. Despite this, the frequency with which confusion creeps into these relationships is notorious. This occurs because we are not dealing with rules, definitions, and procedures, but with human beings who, despite their degree of sophistication, fortunately continue to function as human beings. That this is the case gives our work whatever efficacy it possesses, but at the same time produces those transference and countertransference distortions which threaten our success.

Though obvious, it perhaps can bear emphasis that the point of intake—that is, the time at which the clinic is contacted either by the family or by the referring agency—is crucial in the further relationship of all three. This initial contact, when understood, may serve to clarify the relationship of family, agency, and clinic and to produce a pooling of effort on a mutual problem. On the other hand, when the intake is improperly handled, endless complications may develop which serve only to befog the issue and threaten the success of whatever work either the agency or the clinic have been doing or may attempt to do with the family. The factors which require understanding and clarification reside not only in the nature of the family's problem, but equally in the nature of the relationship between all three participants.

In some cases the referring agency may call the intake worker of the clinic on the phone to discuss the referral, and a report of the agency's work with the patient may be sent either before or after the patient is seen in the clinic. (The term "patient" is here used to refer to the member of the family who makes the initial application.) The phone conversation may be useful, and the report may provide an excellent review of what the agency has learned about the patient; nevertheless, there is at times little more than a hint of the actual circumstances which led up to the clinic referral, or what the agency has actually experienced with the patient. On such occasions the clinic obtains only the vaguest idea of the specific problem or problems the agency, in terms of its own organization and function, was facing with the patient. Thus the agency may not have specifically defined the help it requires, nor will the clinic have clarified for the agency just what it can offer in helping toward the solution of the problem which the agency is facing.

The agency, from its viewpoint, feels perfectly clear in the conviction that one or more members of the family require psychotherapy. The intake worker, while ready to accept the agency's views as a starting point, listens to the patient's story for one or two interviews, evaluates his problems in terms of the clinic's philosophy and organization, and may arrive at a somewhat different conclusion. The problem has been presented by the agency and understood by the clinic in terms of one or more members of a given family requiring psychotherapy. It is presented as a request that the clinic, by the "magical" means of psychotherapy, change the attitude of a patient so that he can better utilize the services of the agency. It is presented as a request that the clinic by the same means change the attitude and behavior of a child so that he becomes more amenable to orthodox educational procedures, or that he desist from breaking the laws of society. It is rarely presented in terms of the impasse arrived at by the agency in providing its characteristic service. The problem the agency itself is facing with the patient in its own work is only secondarily referred to, if mentioned at all.

Beside the factor already suggested as contributing to this situation, there are at least two other important factors—perhaps they are really one. The first of these is that the patient often presents a somewhat different view of his problem to the clinic intake worker, particularly regarding the events leading up to the referral. This may be due in large part to the fact that the intake worker sees the patient only a few times, often only once, and thus is not able to obtain as clear a picture as that possessed by the agency. The other factor is the opportunity presented to the patient for an expression of his ambivalent feelings toward the agency by subtle distortions and misquotations, none necessarily intentional.

There are probably other factors as well, and at some time it would be worthwhile to elaborate further on those already mentioned. The important point, however, is that a situation is created where a difference of opinion or a conflict can, and often does, develop between the referring agency and the clinic. Since the two frequently do not meet, the difference of opinion is often expressed through the patient. This again presents a temptation for the already strong ambivalences of the patient to gain expression by the accentuation and distortion of the differences.

THE QUESTION OF READINESS FOR THERAPY

Conflict between the agency and the clinic at the point of intake may often be expressed over the question of the readiness or the suitability of the family for psychotherapy. The agency may feel quite firm in its conviction that the family is ready for such work and has been adequately prepared for the referral. From the viewpoint of the agency's experiences with the family, this is no doubt thoroughly valid. Despite this, however, by the time the applying parent is seen by the clinic intake worker (the time interval is probably an important factor), he may find himself facing a patient who is extraordinarily ambivalent about therapy, fearful of its nature, derogated by its vague and mysterious implications; notwith-standing the earnest explanations of the intake worker, the patient may in the initial interview or shortly thereafter make it quite clear that he is not at all interested in psychotherapy and would like to forget the whole business. The worker may struggle—usually with little success—to convince the patient of the clinic's potential usefulness in his particular problem; or he may help the patient withdraw his application with minimal consideration of what further action, other than psychotherapy, the patient may be ready to take in solving the problem. He may now feel that the referring agency has been wrong in its judgment regarding the patient's need for psychiatric help and that the problems of the patient and his family could be adequately handled in the agency setting, if only they had a better grasp of the problem. He may even harbor the suspicion that the agency used some form of subtle, and perhaps not so subtle, pressure in guiding the patient to the clinic, particu-larly if the agency has some legal authority, such as a court, or if the agency is providing some form of supplementary help. These feelings, rarely openly expressed (they may not even be in the full awareness of the intake worker), may nevertheless gain expression and be communicated through the various contacts that one worker has with the other. The patient is an excellent medium for their expression and transmission, in addition to which his sensing of them serves to support and accentuate his own ambivalence.

The agency worker, hearing of the fate of his carefully consid-ered plan, may feel disappointed, and this feeling will be accentu-ated by his concern over whatever difficulties led to the referral. He feels that he has carefully evaluated the indications for refer-ring the patient to the clinic, and that he has been most painstaking and thorough in preparing the patient for this step. He may even suspect that through ineptness or for some other reason the clinic worker has in some manner sabotaged his work. Thus, resentment toward the clinic develops in the agency worker, and by communi-cation, in other workers in the agency. By repetition of such epi-sodes the agency begins to feel that the clinic is not of much help in its problems. It rarely happens that the differences and result-ing feelings are ever expressed openly between the two parties to the conflict. In discussions between them the differences and the associated feelings are usually concealed, expressed only indirectly, or projected on the patient. One agency worker, when informed by telephone that a patient whom he had referred to the clinic had de-cided not to continue with the plan for psychotherapy, remarked with evident irritation, "I am disgusted with people whom I try to get in-to therapy and who then refuse to accept the help." It is perhaps unnecessary to point out that such a statement reflects his irritation not only with the patient but at least in part with the clinic as well.

AMBIVALENCE IN PATIENTS AND AGENCIES

It will be useful to consider in greater detail some of the more obvious factors which contribute to the development of this situation. In discussing his problem with the clinic intake worker, the patient may in some way indicate a feeling that he had little inclination to apply for psychotherapeutic help, and was pressured into applying to the clinic. This may be true even though he had accepted the agency worker's suggestion willingly and even enthusiastically at the outset. Such ambivalence is probably present to some extent in all patients, and in this specific situation may indicate some still unresolved feelings toward the referring person. When the patient has been, or still is, dependent upon the referring agency for some benefits, such as supplementation of income, payments for a foster child, or providing some form of care for a natural child (medical care or education), this may be particularly true.

The personality of the intake worker and the degree of his understanding of the dynamic forces operating in this situation become of vital importance in determining the solution of the problem now facing him. His ability to make the necessary discriminations in his feelings toward the patient and the referring agency, as well as the clarity with which he understands the role of the referring agency, that of the clinic, and how they are related, both in the similarity and dissimilarity of their functions, will influence the further handling of the contact. Because of the natural tendency we all have to identify with the patient, the focus of the worker's attention may be diverted from the problem for which he was referred to the fruitless consideration of the patient's open or veiled complaints of coercion.

It is important for the intake worker to make a synthesis between the therapeutically essential attitude of listening to the patient with respect, recognizing and accepting the patient's feelings whatever they may be, and the careful scrutiny of the reality which seems to have evoked these feelings. Without offering interpretations, he must keep in mind the degree of the transference implications of these complaints. At the same time he needs to recognize and openly acknowledge the realistic core of the patient's complaints. This need not involve joining in the attack on the referring agency, which is implicitly or at least potentially an attack on the clinic as well.

When the patient is actually receiving benefits from the referring agency, as mentioned before, or when the agency is a court or other legal authority, the realistic element of coercion cannot be ignored. This is true even though the referral is honestly made as a suggestion for further help, and the agency has no intention of utilizing its coercive power. A patient concerned about possible punitive measures directed at him, or about the possible loss of any one of a number of services essential to him, would hesitate to ignore such advice even when it is sincerely given without any coercive intent. In this respect, the intake worker can only recognize frankly with the patient the reality of the situation. It is necessary in addition, however, to examine thoroughly with him the known facts of the problem for which he was referred.

The nature of the relationship of the clinic to the referring source must also be recognized, and points of identity, as well as boundaries of function, must be very clearly defined for the patient. This is certainly important when the clinic is part of a legal institution or works very closely with it in an advisory capacity. If the function of such a clinic is primarily diagnostic, this becomes of even greater importance, since the brevity of the contact with the patient does not permit the adequate working through of the natural suspicions and fears which preoccupy him. At the same time, the essentially passive, non-manipulative role of the clinic must receive at least a preliminary statement. This requires essentially a clear but simple statement of the nature of psychotherapy, with a particular emphasis on the boundaries of function. The latter underlines the fact that regardless of the coercion, real or imagined, placed on the patient to attend regular interviews, the ability of a therapist to help is in large part directly proportional to the real desire of the patient for psychotherapeutic help. Even with faithful attendance at interviews, the patient is still in a position to frustrate all the efforts of the clinic to help him. Therapeutic help can only be offered—it cannot be forced upon anyone. At least it can go no further than clarifying for both the patient and the clinic that psychotherapeutic help with his problems is not wanted, or cannot be utilized. Even this should not be considered a negligible result for a brief contact.

The real feelings of a patient toward referral for psychotherapy may not become evident until the referral is actually realized. The specific method used in referral is also important. Against this background the ambivalences of the patient are often dramatically outlined. When the worker in the referring agency, as a part of good social work procedure, "helps" the patient by calling the clinic and making an appointment, he is often dismayed to discover later that the appointment was not kept. Even when the patient takes the initiative in making his own appointment, all sorts of difficulties may develop. Every hour offered him by the clinic interferes with some other "important" activity. Finally, when an hour is decided upon, sometimes at some inconvenience to the intake worker, the patient may later call and cancel, perhaps asking for another appointment. Even then he may fail or cancel, following which there is an exchange of letters and phone calls which may or may not end in an appointment being made and kept. Thus a great deal of time and emotional energy is spent around the issue of an appointment, which only serves to encourage the patient's tendency to express his ambivalences by such acting-out. The sooner both the referring agency and the clinic grasp the significance of these seemingly realistic difficulties in making an appointment, the sooner they will begin to evaluate with the patient what he is really ready to do about his problem.

Another point at which a patient may be referred to a clinic is when his worker at the agency is leaving. The reasons for this reside not only in the nature of the patient's problem but even more in the state of the relationship between patient and worker at the time. It may be a manifestation of what is probably anxiety over separation, shared by both, which for a variety of reasons has not been sufficiently worked through. In one such case the worker who was leaving an agency was extremely anxious to have a patient accepted at the clinic. There were many phone calls and exchanges of letters, and the patient was finally accepted for treatment. The patient had not yet been assigned to a therapist when it was found necessary to contact the agency for some additional information. The new worker at the agency had not yet become acquainted with the patient, who was part of his case load, and apparently was not aware that he had been referred to the clinic by his predecessor. While not actively opposed to referral, he suggested that he would like to acquaint himself with the patient and his problem before any further steps were taken. The new worker ultimately did not find it necessary to refer the patient, and the case was closed in the clinic.

Occasionally situations occur where a worker, upon leaving the agency, attempts to refer an adolescent to a clinic with little or no consultation with his parents regarding the referral, or where the readiness of the parents for such referral has been insufficiently considered. In one such instance, an adolescent boy who had been followed for some time in a school counseling service was referred when his worker was about to leave the agency. The worker was extremely anxious that this referral be accepted, made several phone calls to the clinic, and finally came in for a conference to urge the acceptance of this boy for treatment. When a question was raised as to the attitude of the parent, in this case the father, the mother being out of the home, it was rather briefly dismissed with the comment that the father was not particularly interested. Since it was clinic policy always to contact the parents, the father was asked to come in for an appointment. He seemed greatly confused and concerned. He expressed surprise that the problem was of a nature that required psychiatric help, but since he had been concerned about his son for a long time, he expressed willingness for the boy to receive such help and was himself willing to participate in regular interviews. Further interviews however, soon revealed that he had felt left out, criticized, and depreciated by the agency.

THE TRIANGLE

Situations may arise in which two separate agencies are involved in helping the patient. Because they have a somewhat different orientation and approach, friction may occur, leading to constantly mounting tension and finally resulting in one or the other referring the patient to the clinic for psychotherapy. This sort of difficulty can frequently occur between a voluntary social agency and a legal agency such as a court. An example of this occurs when an agency is given the direct responsibility for the placement of a child who is at the same time a ward of the court. The agency is interested in finding a placement which will be most conducive to the child's welfare and happiness. The court, on the other hand, must also be cognizant of certain legalities, such as the existence of relatives who may be required to accept responsibility for care, residence requirements, financial obligations of the various governmental units, and other such considerations. Strict attention to these details by the court may threaten a placement which the agency feels is particularly desirable for the child. Unable perhaps to gain its point with the court, or in anxious anticipation of such failure even before negotiations between the two have taken place, the agency may refer the child for psychotherapy, emphasizing to the clinic the degree of emotional disturbance in the child. The real reason for the referral, which is the hope that the clinic will support the agency in its conflict with the court, may hardly be mentioned or come out only indirectly.

CASE ILLUSTRATION

The following example illustrates what may occur during the intake process between the clinic and another agency also interested in the patient. Mrs. B. applied to the clinic on her own initiative for help with her nine-year-old son, who was difficult to manage both at home and at school. In the first interview she signed a permit allowing the clinic to obtain information from the school but asked the worker to wait at least two weeks before sending for a school report. She explained that the school was prejudiced against her and her son, and she wanted the worker to become acquainted with her first. When reminded two weeks later, she again asked her worker to refrain from contacting the school. She led the worker to believe that the school knew nothing about her application to the clinic.

However, the day after this interview the principal of the school called and asked for information about the clinic's work with the family. The intake worker, surprised by this call, became quite anxious, having in mind the mother's wish that the school not know about her application, and tried to explain to the principal the clinic's inability to give out any information without permission from the patient. The principal became angry and with frank irritation announced that she had received permission from Mrs. B. to obtain this information and named accurately the time and day when Mrs. B. was seen at the clinic. The worker, completely defensive at this point, continued to say that he had had only a few contacts with the family, that he had very little information at this point, that what he had would probably not be very useful to the school, but that he would be glad to have the school get in touch with him later when he would have had an opportunity for a more thorough evaluation of the problem. This seemed to infuriate the principal even more, and the conversation ended on this note with the worker thoroughly uneasy about his management of the conversation.

Several weeks later the principal called again, this time talking to the therapist assigned to the child. She again asked for information regarding the problem, at the same time pointing out the difficulties she was having with the child, and asked for suggestions about his management. The therapist felt uneasy at these incessant demands for information and advice, and fearful that what he might say would involve a breach of confidence, tended to be somewhat evasive in his discussion. This angered the principal even more, and she rejected the therapist's offer of a conference, saying that since the clinic didn't offer any information or advice, she didn't see the usefulness of a conference. After a discussion with the consultant regarding the nature of the situation and the issues involved, the therapist phoned the principal, admitting that he had probably not been very helpful, that he had not clearly understood the problem she was facing, and suggested a conference to discuss the various issues in the case, as well as those between the school and the clinic.

At the conference the principal spent a great deal of time criticizing child guidance clinics, psychiatrists, and social workers, particularly for their secretiveness and lack of helpfulness in school problems. This was all accepted without comment. She then related her experience with the child and his mother, expressing her impatience with both and pointing to all her efforts to help them, and then indirectly indicated curiosity about what the mother was saying about the school and whether the mother was blaming her for the child's difficulties. It soon became clear that the immediate problem was the principal's feelings of helplessness and defeat in her efforts to help the child and anxiety that she might even cause harm. She needed to share her difficulties with someone able to reassure her in the specific work she had to do with both parent and child.

Similar problems tend to arise during the progress of therapy when an agency continues to function in some aspect of a patient's life, or when it is drawn in by the patient for help with a specific problem. An outstanding instance of this occurs in foster home care when the agency continues to have basic responsibility for supervision. Under these circumstances the agency social worker usually continues periodically to see the foster mother as well as the child. While this is probably necessary, it does present an opportunity for the unresolved ambivalences of any or all of the participants to gain expression in some subtle form difficult to recognize and even more difficult to deal with. This very fact, however, can seriously threaten the success of the work each is attempting to do. The potential number of triangular tension situations is limited only by the number of people participating in the work.

The foster mother may resent the agency social worker and feel that the worker is exercising too much control over her management of the child. This resentment is perhaps always present, though rarely consciously perceived, even though the worker is quite clear regarding her role in relation to both the child and the foster mother, and actually does not attempt management under the guise of support. Often the worker may react rather strongly to some of the foster mother's attitudes, and, without openly expressing her disagreement, may try by indirect means to modify her management of the child. Usually each has mixed feelings, combining varying proportions of hostility and guilt. For this reason they are not clearly apprehended and rarely come to direct expression. Instead they are expressed in subtly distorted ways, attached to apparently valid observations and complaints, and tend to be acted out, frequently in relation to the child. Each may then attempt to draw the clinic therapist into the unexpressed conflict as a presumably neutral referee but actually in an attempt to gain an ally.

In the following instance the competitive and resentful feelings of the foster mother toward the agency social worker were fairly clear. The social worker had made plans to take the child on an outing in celebration of his birthday. When she came to the home to meet the boy, the foster mother informed her that the boy had behaved badly recently, and as a punishment she had withdrawn her

permission for the outing. The worker felt that, since she had
promised the boy this outing and since he had looked forward to it
with keen anticipation, she would have to keep her promise. Here
we have the sharpening of a conflict in a triangular situation in
which there is a grave risk of the child becoming the medium
through whom the conflict is expressed. At the same time this
presents the child with an opportunity for exploiting the mounting
tensions between the social worker and the foster mother by acting
out some of his own ambivalent feelings. Thus we have all the conditions which may gradually or rapidly lead to the point where complete disruption will occur—usually around a realistic and manifest-
ly valid point. This may result in the removal of the child from the
home with all the traumatic possibilities that the periodic repetition
of such separations entail for the child.

The foster mother's therapist at the clinic was drawn into this
conflict, thus creating another triangular constellation, which included the agency social worker, the foster mother, and the therapist.
The therapist became the focus for the ambivalent feelings of the
other two. The real source of the conflict was neither openly expressed nor clearly indicated, but was latently present in the complaints of both. The foster mother expressed it in her skepticism
regarding the need or usefulness of psychotherapy for the child.
She felt imposed on by both the agency and the clinic in that they
expected her to bring the child to the clinic. She felt that she was
quite capable of managing his behavior, and failed to see any serious
emotional problems in the child as they were presented to her by the
agency worker.

The conflict was further accentuated by the requirement of the
clinic that she also participate through regular interviews with a
worker at the clinic. She presented all kinds of ostensibly valid
reasons why regular weekly attendance at the clinic was not possible. She frequently failed to keep or canceled appointments and often
came late to those that she did keep. Without obvious intent she
promoted and exploited differences between the agency worker and
the clinic therapist, complaining to one about the other. On one
occasion the agency worker was present when the foster mother was
preparing to take the boy to the clinic for his regular appointment.
She pointedly exhibited a bouquet of flowers to the worker which she
intended as a gift to her clinic worker. She did not make any similar
presentation to the agency worker.

In view of the work being attempted at the clinic with both foster
mother and child, the agency worker felt uneasy and uncertain about
her specific role with this foster mother. Her own unconscious
tendency toward competition with the clinic worker, stimulated by
whatever frustrations she was experiencing in her own work with

the mother, probably played an important part in increasing the tensions between all three. Under these circumstances an agency worker may feel that the clinic worker is not doing a good job in teaching the foster mother how to help the child and perhaps is putting obstacles in the way of her own efforts to do so. The clinic worker, on the other hand, may tend to identify too much with the foster mother, possibly in part because of her own unconscious competitiveness with the agency worker, and may feel that the latter is interfering more than warranted in the relationship between the foster mother and the child. She may further feel that this interference is impeding the smooth progress of therapy. Thus, a situation may occur in which, without any of the participants being clearly aware of it, the clinic worker may subtly support the defiant tendencies of the mother toward the agency worker, and the latter may unconsciously strengthen the mother's resistance to therapy. The result may be a premature closure of the case.

The unconscious tendency in the patient to play one agency off against another is clearly brought out in the case of a nine-year-old child who refused to go to school because of severe nausea when he was in the classroom. The mother and child were referred to the clinic by the guidance division of the public schools. The mother felt it would be cruel to force the child to attend school and wanted a home teacher assigned until "the treatment would take effect." The school required a written statement from the clinic stating that a home teacher was necessary to safeguard the child's health. The clinic, working with both mother and child, felt that this would defeat the ends of therapy by stressing the invalidism of the child and thereby graphically expressing doubt about the capacity of both mother and child to resolve their problem with each other.

The mother made a great issue of a home teacher, with the worker at the guidance services as well as with her therapist at the clinic. It soon became clear that in addition to whatever validity there was in this request for a home teacher, the mother was using it as a form of resistance at a point when she was coming closer to an awareness of her own ambivalent relationship to the child. At the same time it became a means of emphasizing and exploiting the differences between the clinic and the guidance services. This was clearly seen at a conference between the two agencies during the course of which it was learned that the mother had reported to her clinic worker that the guidance services insisted that the clinic doctor sign the permit for a home teacher. However, to the worker at the guidance services she had reported only that the clinic simply refused to sign the permit under any circumstances. As a result the conference began with the workers from both agencies feeling rather uneasy and tense in each other's presence. It was only when the mother's statement to each was brought out, and discussed in the light of the operation of each agency, that the tension was resolved, and progress was then made in defining their respective roles in helping the mother and child to use their services constructively.

In this paper I have not been concerned specifically with the symptoms in the child or in the mother, or the psychological history of either one which led to the development of the presenting symptoms. The problems referred to in this paper are essentially transference and countertransference in nature and stem from the particular psychological history of all the participants. Their understanding and resolution lies in focusing attention not only on the child's experiences nor even on the subtleties of his relationship to the significant adults in his environment. They require rather that the major focus be on the nature and development of the relationship between the family, or the applying adult in that family, and the various agencies and individuals who are drawn in to help resolve a problem. Constant, close attention to the manifest aspects of these relationships can lead to an increasing understanding of the latent content, the unconscious forces operating, and the subtleties which are not altogether in the full awareness of any or all the participants. In this way the surprising and frustrating difficulties which develop may ultimately lend themselves to understanding and may then be dealt with psychologically with relative precision, thus permitting the therapeutic job to proceed constructively.

This does not mean that further difficulties will not occur. These are to be expected as a natural concomitant of such work, just as resistances are part and parcel of individual work. When viewed in this fashion these difficulties can be seen not merely as annoying nuisances but rather as useful material which can be put to a constructive use in elucidating and understanding the problem of the specific family.

SUGGESTED ADDITIONAL READINGS

1. FREUD, A. Psychoanalytical treatment of children. London; Imago Pub. Co., 1947.

2. STANTON, A. H., & SCHWARTZ, M. S. The management of a type of institutional participation in mental illness. Psychiatry, 12:13, 1949.

3. STANTON, A. H., & SCHWARTZ, M. S. Observations on dissociation as social participation. Psychiatry, 12:339, 1949.

4. SZUREK, S. A. Some problems in collaborative therapy. News-Letter, Am. Assoc. of Psychiat. Soc. Work., 9:4, 1940.

5. SZUREK, S. A., JOHNSON, A. M., & FALSTEIN, E. I. Collaborative psychiatric therapy of parent-child problems. Am. J. Orthopsychiat., 12:3, 1942. Reprinted in S. A. Szurek and I. N. Berlin (Eds.), Training in therapeutic work with children. Vol. 2, the Langley Porter Child Psychiatry Series. Palo Alto, Calif.: Science and Behavior Books, 1967.

6. WHITAKER, C. A., WARKENTIN, J., & JOHNSON, N. The psychotherapeutic impasse. Am. J. Orthopsychiat., 20:641, 1950.

SECTION FOUR

THE COURTS, THE CHILD PSYCHIATRIST, AND THE ANTISOCIAL CHILD

INTRODUCTION

The role of juvenile courts in dealing with the delinquent has always been an important one, although in many instances ineffective. An increasing realization of how the child psychiatrist and insight from psychiatric concepts can augment the effectiveness of juvenile probation work has resulted in the collaborative efforts which are described in the following papers.

INTERRELATIONSHIP OF THE CORRECTIONAL WORKER, THE OFFENDER, AND THE LEGAL STRUCTURE*

Samuel Susselman

While the chief effort of the community in devising a legal structure to deal with the offender is to safeguard itself, implicit in such a structure is the intention of rehabilitating the offender to take his place in society without special restrictions. There are exceptions, of course, in those individuals who have so threatened society by their behavior that the constituted authorities, supported by the laws and their right to interpret the laws, forbid these individuals to return to the community. These individuals are sentenced to life imprisonment or death. All other proven transgressors either are given an opportunity to remain in the community under probation, or, after confinement, are released on parole. The ultimate objective appears to be the eventual removal of all special controls such as probation and parole. The role of the correctional worker, if he is to carry out the intent of the community, appears to be twofold: law enforcement, and rehabilitation of the individual.

The twofold nature of this role is more apparent than real, however. It might be more correct to say that the function of probation and of parole is to rehabilitate the individual, and enforcement of the laws constitutes part of this corrective process.

As a psychiatrist considering the process of rehabilitation, I feel obliged to begin by considering those manifestations of antisocial behavior that are expressions of emotional conflict—the only manifestations about which I feel I have any right to speak. They may not encompass the entire range of antisocial conduct, but I believe that many antisocial acts fall into the category of neurotic behavior. In this case any successful effort at rehabili-

---

*This paper was delivered at the Fourth Annual Training Institute for Probation, Parole, and Institutional Staff, University of California, Berkeley, August 8, 1962.

tation must be concerned with the causes of the disturbed behavior, with the offender's conflicts and their resolution. The correctional worker's emotional involvements, when they occur, are also obstacles whose reduction will facilitate the process of rehabilitation. If we are to assume that we can help to modify an individual's emotional pattern, we must assume first that the pattern is modifiable—that it is not inherited, but acquired. It is not farfetched to assume that emotional conflict was acquired in an atmosphere of emotional conflict. We cannot be helpful to others in those moments when we are in conflict ourselves. I cannot hope to convince those of you who are not already convinced of this simple thesis—that anxiety begets anxiety—I can only state my conviction of its validity. As will become apparent, it is alternately the main theme or the background for much of what I have to say.

PURPOSE OF LEGAL STRUCTURE

The legal structure is an instrument, devised by those members of a community who have achieved authority, to regulate the activities of the community. An extreme example of this is an autocracy, in which one individual is in sole command. In a democracy it is understood that the individuals in authority are committed to conform to the same regulations that they formulate for others. At any one moment the legal structure may be regarded as a progressively evolving institution with a long history and an unpredictable future. It consists of the residues from the authorities of the past modified by the authorities of the present. Since in a democracy final authority resides in the majority of the community, those elected or appointed to legal authority are limited in their right to make changes. The moment a legal authority assumes office he is bound both by the formulations of the past and by the authority of the community in the present. Therefore, the quality and type of modifications in the devices of the legal structure—namely, the laws—depends on the quality of the people in legal authority and the quality of the people in the community. Any changes in the spirit of the laws depend on the amount of time it takes to alter the spirit of the people. Since the authorities of the past are dead and the authorities of the future are unborn, we can deal only with ourselves, some of the present authorities, in order to improve on our inheritance. We can select those things that after careful examination seem valid for us. We can add to our legacy whatever results from the increased clarity of thinking we may each of us achieve in his own lifetime, reflecting the changing influences to which we are exposed in our generation. In an attempt to achieve this end, let us then examine certain concepts and situations.

AUTHORITY-SUBORDINATE RELATIONSHIPS

The direction of responsibility in authority-subordinate relationships usually is clearly expressed and accepted in discussions of these relationships: the subordinate is responsible to the authority. The authority holds the subordinate responsible, especially when the subordinate cannot or will not hold himself responsible. We recognize this as an important thesis, from which the concept of limits and the manner in which limits are applied have been derived. We recognize that emotional benefits accrue when limits are consistently and maturely applied; that the punitively-used limits can call forth rebellion in the subordinate; and that vacillation in the setting of limits encourages in the subordinate behavior that is detrimental to himself and to others.

What has not been clear to me until recently, naive as it may sound, is the subordinate position that is occupied by every authority in a democracy. Even top authority is subordinate to the community and to the legal structure. Each successive rank of authority is responsible to the rank above him. Thus, every authority and every subordinate occupies a midway position between a subordinate and a superior in the hierarchy. Eventually, this becomes a circular process that can be formulated in the following way. The legal structure is responsible to the community; the community is responsible to the legal structure. The basic, modifiable units in both the legal structure and the community are individuals. Every individual is at the same time an authority and a subordinate, carrying in his personality the results of his interpersonal relations with individuals in the community. To study such a situation in its entirety is difficult and defeating. However, an examination of certain aspects of this circular system may lead to some understanding of the whole.

LAW: THE LIMITS SET BY SOCIETY

My speculations lead me to state that a law does not come into existence unless it is thought to be necessary. It becomes necessary when certain circumstances or anticipated circumstances disturb the level of comfort that a community enjoys. The lawmakers are charged by the community with the responsibility for at least restoring the former level of comfort. Often this can be done simply and easily. Crime, especially, produces a high degree of discomfort. The lawmaker may feel less discomfort than the community, and he may see that there is little or no cause for the discomfort; but because of the large number of people involved and the diversity of pressures, the lawmaker has little opportunity to inquire fully into the reason for community discomfort with the intention of allaying it without passing a law.

In certain instances a lawmaker may stand firm against taking action or may trust to the passage of time for the discomfort to subside, at least in his legal colleagues. But often the lawmaker is expected to respond promptly to the demands of a public aroused by the acts of deviant individuals. The quality and terms of the eventual legislation reflect the degree of concern stirred up in the lawmakers thus under pressure. For example, after a series of vicious sex crimes the public demands extremely punitive measures, but these demands gradually diminish in intensity as matters are discussed and concern lessens. The laws that are finally formulated are intended not only to restore the comfort of the community but also to restore comfort to the pressured lawmaker. Again, the terms of the new laws are dictated by the degree of concern felt at the time of ratification—the more concerned the lawmaker, the more severe the terms and restrictions. Unfortunately, such laws, once they are codified and passed, remain relatively static. They may be regarded as the lawmaker's way of protecting himself from further concern and of discharging his responsibility to the community. Whatever we may say or feel about these laws, they represent the best solution for regulating the functioning of the community that the lawmakers can contrive at any one moment. Whatever the laws, their violation has the potential of re-creating concern in the lawmaker and the community.

One can demonstrate that a judge's decision is made in much the same manner. Some decisions are arrived at easily, simply, and so obviously that they allow of no disagreement. Other decisions are made in an atmosphere of concern, and their terms may be severe and punitive, depending upon the degree of concern in the particular judge. That is why, under similar laws, decisions will vary from county to county and from judge to judge. As with the laws, a decision once made cannot be disregarded without potentially re-creating concern in the judge. Similarly, one can analyze the circumstances under which the policy of the administrator comes into being, e.g., the definition of the function of the correctional worker. Once these concepts and methods are formulated, they tend to become operational tools which, if disregarded, particularly by subordinates in the hierarchal structure, re-create concern in the authority held responsible. The subordinate at any level in the hierarchy, unless he has ready access to, and full communication with, his immediate superior, has no way of knowing which policy he can safely bypass. (Actually, he has no authority to do so at all.) In these circumstances he has no choice but to conform, despite his disagreements, to whichever of the tools he may be using (regulations, laws, decisions, or policies) unless he is released from conformity and from responsibility by his superior. Otherwise, he risks arousing concern in himself, for he in turn will be held accountable to others.

The formalized basis of the legal structure is the law, which is relatively rigid. The people who can alter the legal structure are the lawmakers, who in practice cannot be influenced by most of us because of time, distance, and lack of personal acquaintance. However, we work not in a framework of laws alone, but also within an inner framework that has certain codified parts called decisions, policies, and functions—to name a few. These too may become rigid, but like the laws they are formulated by people subject to the same kind of pressures and anxieties as are the lawmakers. These are the people with whom we deal every day. They and we are the fluctuating, dynamic, fluid components that constitute a still more central framework, one that is more readily modifiable and with which we can deal face to face.

I have attempted briefly to translate the legal structure concerned with crime into components—not only what has been codified as laws, decisions, policies, and functions, but also people, for we can deal with people. We can recognize from the previous discussion that what we enforce are not always the laws as originally formulated, but rather elements that have been derived from the laws, filtered and colored by passage through various individuals in the hierarchy of authority, until, by the time they reach the client, they sometimes cannot be recognized. We must, therefore, consider the people working in the legal situation and the tools that the legal structure has produced for their use. All of these tools represent limits which, if violated or by-passed, may beget anxieties in every direction. The work of rehabilitation is hampered if anxiety is present in people at various levels of the hierarchy of authority.

Limits are not peculiar to legal settings. Problems of authority and of limits are present at home, in the schools, at work, etc. When it comes to the legal structure I think we can agree that: (1) laws are necessary for people in our society; (2) laws are intended to define limits beyond which an individual cannot go without disturbing the comfort of the community; and (3) there should be individuals in the community with the delegated responsibility to see that these limits are enforced.

There is probably little that I can tell you about the proper application of limits that you do not already know; you may have observed many times that setting limits is one of the factors in the rehabilitation of a social deviant. You have seen what happens when hostilely aggressive youths, who get into all kinds of difficulties in the community, are placed in custody. Having been unable to set proper limits for themselves, they often feel relieved when someone puts an end to their uneasy, self-destructive behavior. The

Heierens boy was a classical example of this (see page 66). If the quality of one's own limits are such that they permit or provoke destructive behavior, which in turn is derived from self-destructive attitudes, proper limits from without are beneficial both to the individual and to the society in which he lives.

But what of so-called "punitive" laws or policies—can we consider them limits that can be helpful? I do not know if I can answer this question to the satisfaction of everyone. I feel, however, that the laws that concern us, in addition to whatever other implications they may contain, do include definite limits.

It is my impression that the incipient offender's behavior developed as it did partly because early in life he was not often enough presented alternative choices by his parents or parental substitutes; or, the alternatives may have been neither timely enough nor unambivilent enough. In other words, if the consequences of a contemplated destructive course of action are made unmistakably clear, some potential offenders might choose to conform rather than to rebel. It is obvious that severely impulsive individuals would disregard any approach, no matter how well presented, unless it is repeated often enough with proper timing and when the consequences of maladaptive behavior have had sufficient emotional impact.

THE DANGER OF NONENFORCEMENT

If the law enforcer takes upon himself the authority to disregard even a punitive law, he automatically does at least these two things, despite the care with which alternatives are identified for him: he disregards the limits set by law, and he appoints himself an unauthorized authority, placing himself above the legal authority. By his own rebellion against the laws of society, he is supporting the transgressor in his rebellion against society. In other words, the alternatives to not enforcing even a punitive law are more damaging to the law enforcer, to society, and, I believe, to the transgressor than is enforcing such a law. Constituted authority is ignored by nonenforcement, and constituted authority will not tolerate this. Limits have been by-passed.

One may suggest another possible and far-reaching result of such disregard for existing laws. Obviously, laws that are not effective must be replaced by others, and these may be even more restrictive than the old laws that the law enforcement officer had disregarded. In that case, the officer who fails to enforce punitive laws is partially responsible for perhaps more stringent and more punitive laws.

Can we arrive at a reasonable solution other than the strict enforcement of distasteful laws? Let us consider incarceration, which is looked upon as a punitive measure by most people. In the hope of being helpful to the offender, one might explain the essence of the measure thus: "We cannot tolerate you in our community, at the moment, because you interfere with our ease and comfort. We are therefore incarcerating you until such time as you can convince us by your behavior and attitude that we can again trust you in our midst." Does not the same thinking hold true of conditions of probation and parole, which some consider punitive, although less so than incarceration? Is not the enforcement officer representing the legal structure by saying, "We cannot trust you (the offender) in our community without some kind of check on your activity and, therefore, we place you under supervision. When you can convince us that you may be trusted without such checks on your activities, we shall remove these restrictions." These essentials, elementary as they may seem, are often lost through distortion; but when communicated clearly, they can certainly produce constructive results. They will hold up against any distortion by the offender. Once we have isolated limits as a basic factor and once we have recognized the importance of maintaining these limits, it may be less difficult to express our feelings and attitudes about punitive overtones. For instance, we may feel free to say, "It is regrettable that our prisons and detention facilities do not meet all your needs, but these are all we have." Or, "Unfortunately, the law as constituted does not allow modification of the period of incarceration. You may be emotionally ready to leave detention sooner than we can allow you to do so under the law." Or, "I, too, disagree with this or that provision, but if you transgress again, we have no other choice." My point is that once we have accepted the limits in the law as a reality and agree with the necessity for enforcing the limits that we have clearly defined, we may then feel free to express our own disagreements with certain parts of the law. Too often the overtones that are considered punitive become confused with the limits proper, and we find ourselves unintentionally disagreeing with the limiting portion of the law.

Surprisingly, problems also may arise with a nonpunitive law. A nonpunitive law, if improperly enforced, may have a punitive result. Let us consider a situation in a different field—that of public health.

Five years ago Mr. Brown, the father of four children, was diagnosed as suffering from tuberculosis. There is a long history of tuberculosis in the family, Mr. Brown's mother having died of the disease when he was thirteen years old. When the diagnosis of tuberculosis was made, the patient, in the interest of himself and of his family, consented to enter a sanatorium. After a short time, he signed himself out against advice and has since refused sanatorium care. The public health nurses report that although Mr. Brown is faithful about visiting the outpatient clinic for treatment, he fails to take adequate precautions in the home and thus exposes his family to infection. Two years ago, a state law was passed that empowered the public health physician to hospitalize such a patient. (Previously, a patient had the right to refuse hospitalization.) Despite this new law, Mr. Brown continued to neglect proper precautions at home, and his wife has since been hospitalized with an active case of tuberculosis with positive sputum (which means she can pass the infection on to other people). Two of his children now have positive tuberculin tests, whereas formerly they were negative. (A positive tuberculin test indicates some degree of infection, but not necessarily a clinical case of the disease.) Even in the face of these developments, Mr. Brown still refused hospitalization, saying that he would go to the hospital only if the police came for him. The nurse tried every possible maneuver to gain his consent to being hospitalized, short of the authority she possesses through her superior officer. She did not want to be the one to "call the police," as she put it. Although it was pointed out to her that she would actually be doing the man, the community, and his family a favor by ordering his hospitalization, she still hesitated to take action. Thus, a nonpunitive measure considered by the nurse to be punitive (i.e., "call the police") resulted in far greater punishment to this family—in the form of a serious illness—by its nonenforcement. Interestingly enough, when Mr. Brown was finally told firmly that he had the alternatives of entering the hospital voluntarily or being brought in by the police, he immediately applied for hospitalization. He has since expressed satisfaction with the decision.

I realize that I have not explained why the nurse thought invoking legal action was punitive; this is a matter of conjecture. My guess is that one of the traditions of the nursing profession is expressed by the statement, "A nurse should be kind, and take care of or relieve suffering." We might also speculate that the nurse felt a need to be a "good fellow." I hope my point is made that a nonpunitive law can have a punitive result if it is not enforced, and that the failure to enforce the limits defined in the laws may lead to serious consequences.

I am sure it is agreed that limits are important, necessary, and helpful if properly applied. Even laws regarded as punitive cannot be overlooked as far as defining limits is concerned. Yet I must be careful, lest what I have been saying be distorted, to stress the fact that the proper application of limits is not a cure-all, and that I am not advocating a "get tough" policy. But when reasonable and mature dealings have succeeded neither in being helpful, nor in putting an end to self-destructive and antisocial behavior, the setting and enforcing of limits has its important and significant place. It is not separate from rehabilitation, but a factor in it.

AUTHORITY, COMPETENCE, AND RESPONSIBILITY

The appointment of an individual to a position of authority carries with it the implication that that individual is competent to discharge the responsibility delegated to him. If the authority, once appointed, succeeds in discharging his responsibility to the satisfaction of those who appointed him, it is assumed that he possesses sufficient competence for the position. In other words, the realistic yardstick for the appointed authority is the appointing authority's evaluation of his discharge of responsibility. Competence is a qualitative thing, difficult to assess directly. It is, therefore, understandable that discharge of responsibility (from the appointing authority's point of view) rather than competence (as evaluated by individuals regarded as experts) becomes the criterion for the success or failure of a person in authority. That is why, for example, statistics are stressed—why quantity (the apparently concrete) assumes greater importance than quality (the apparently intangible)—and why it is important that authority and expert educate each other progressively toward more shared points of view.

The establishment of an authority-subordinate relationship seems to lay the groundwork for distortion. We tend to forget that the designation of a person as a superior usually delegates one accountable thing to him, and that is responsibility—superior responsibility as compared to the subordinate. The delegation of superior responsibility does not necessarily, and cannot always, include superior competence. Distortion, when present, may occur on both sides. On one side, the superior assumes that his competence must be superior to that of his subordinate. Once he has assumed this, he must assert his superior competence regardless of the degree of competence shown by his subordinate. The subordinate gets trapped in the reverse manner. If the subordinate, because of self-depreciation, assumes that his superior should have superior competence at all times, he detects and is quick to exploit any evidence of incompetence, usually by his attitudes since he does not dare to point out the error, feeling as hostile as he does because of his own self-belittling attitudes. If the superior attempts to maintain his fancied position of omniscience, the implied criticism spurs him on to even further efforts to support his untenable position. He is more likely to behave as though he were omniscient, is often punitive, and commits further irrationalities in order to preserve his pretense. This the subordinate exploits still further by rebellious attitudes or by hostile acquiescence and sabotage, which in turn drives the superior to retaliation. And so they go around and around: constructive communication between the two all but ceases, and meeting each other becomes a matter of avoidance of issues.

An authority who always feels perfectly secure—and probably none such exists—would recognize all the factors involved in any situation. He would be quick to know when matters were beyond his own competence but within the range of a subordinate's. For instance, the business executive admits that he knows less than his engineers, or than any of his technicians, about their particular field. The judge delegates most of the work of investigation and supervision of the offender to the probation officer; he will accept recommendations from schools, psychiatrists, and psychologists, and asks to be instructed and educated. A probation officer knows more about most of his own cases than does his supervisor. A parole officer is in a better position to know a parolee than is the parole board. Indeed, the supervisor, the parole board, and the judge generally accept recommendations from their subordinates.

The degree to which the authority can delegate responsibility without concern depends upon his own feeling of security and his ability to relate with both his subordinates and his superiors. The extent to which the subordinate can accept responsibility without concern depends upon his own feeling of security and his ability to relate to others in the hierarchy. Superior responsibility and superior competence do not always go hand in hand. This must be recognized but not exploited.

If the superior does not feel that he must be the most competent in all matters at all times, he can accept disagreement from subordinates in areas in which he is less competent. If the subordinate has respect for his own competence, he can disagree with his superior without challenging him, and thus may contribute to his own feelings of accomplishment and self-respect. Gaining in self-respect is a slow process. It requires interchanges between the self-depreciating individual and another individual less self-depreciating at crucial, anxiety-fraught moments. Such interchanges occur wherever people work together, and many relationships between friends serve this purpose. The system of supervision explicitly embodies this concept. When individuals in a group of two or more become so emotionally involved with each other that an impasse occurs, an increase in the ability of each to view the problem objectively, and new increments in self-respect, may have to come from an uninvolved individual, often someone outside the specific situation. That is why, in any organization, a colleague from another division may at times be more helpful than an immediate supervisor; why a supervisor can be helpful when a judge and a probation officer are at loggerheads; why a probation officer may be helpful in clarifying a crisis in a marital situation; why an administrator may step in to clarify an issue; why a consultant, not subject to existing pressures, may be helpful; why in-service training geared specifically to the relief of anxiety, rather than being wholly devoted to didactic teaching, is often fruitful.

I have attempted to discuss, in a general way, the emotional factors that lie behind the evolution of certain codifications in the legal structure and why these formulations seem necessary, especially those that result from an effort to avoid anxiety and that tend to re-create anxiety when disregarded. I have said something about distortions that occur in evaluations of responsibility and competence. You will understand my reluctance to delve into self-attitudes here, for example, why an enforcement officer at times does not abide by the limits that he can logically recognize as being valid. Any point of contact between two individuals in which distortions may arise deserves study. It is interesting that the subject of study becomes depersonalized in the process and then everything is discussed, except the individuals involved. That is why we study the concept of limits, and not the reason why limits fail to be observed; why we discuss recommendations to the court, and not what is involved for the individuals making recommendations; why we discuss adoptions versus foster home care, institutional placement versus remaining at home, or marriage versus divorce. To do otherwise may evoke threatening emotions. A psychiatrist seeks to deal only with those matters for which the other person is ready—insofar as the psychiatrist can evaluate that readiness, whether that person is a patient or someone from another profession seeking consultation. The psychiatrist also must be emotionally ready. He must abide by the terms of his contract with the participants, a contract that he especially must assist in evolving.

DISTORTIONS IN HIERARCHICAL RELATIONSHIPS

Let us look briefly at one situation in which distortions can occur, namely the making of recommendations to the court by a probation officer. Many things may take place during this procedure. If a distortion enters at the moment of recommendation (and I am not considering the rule, but the exception), further distortions seem to be inevitable. If you will recall the previous discussion of competence, you will recognize the superior-subordinate relationship that exists in this situation. The same factors may exist in a supervisor-worker, or administrator-supervisor relationship.

Advances in probation and parole work have been rapid in the last few years. In addition to developments in the field itself, the thinking of related professions such as sociology, psychology, and psychiatry have become integrated into its philosophies. Indeed, active participation with these professions is becoming the rule, and it is accepted and encouraged by the legal profession. At the present time it is hard to know where probation work stops and casework begins. In many localities the two are identical. It is also hard to know where casework ends and psychotherapy begins; the difference between casework and psychotherapy is a currently debated question. The probation officer is armed with an arsenal of new information and spurred on by the enthusiasm and optimism that fresh insights bring. In addition, he is often identified with his client. If he feels that a certain judge will rule in a certain stereotyped way about a certain type of case, the formulation of the presentation to the judge, though containing all the facts, may be colored with an attitude (I exaggerate, for emphasis) that says, "This is the cold dope, you old fogey." How will the judge react when he gets an intuitive whiff of this attitude on the part of the probation officer? I think you know the answer. His competence is being challenged by derogation; to defend it he is driven to disagree with the probation officer and disregard the recommendation. In the final analysis it is the offender, on the receiving end of the decision, rather than the probation officer who is the victim. Hardly realizing his own role in the situation, the probation officer regards the judge as arbitrary and hostile.

Sometimes, more subtle means are used to slant the evidence and influence the decision. The temptation is great because the judge often accepts the recommendations of the probation officer. However, many consequences are possible. At the moment of presentation, the probation officer may fear that the judge will detect his maneuvering. If he does, the probation officer is on the spot. Even if the judge does not, both he and the probation officer may know, in some vague way, that something not clearly communicated is going on. This not only makes for a poor working relationship and impairs further dealings between the two, but has other consequences as well. In effect, the probation officer takes upon himself the role of the judge. The recommendation becomes the decision because the judge takes the probation officer's recommendation. If the recommendation is a lenient one, compared to the judge's anticipated decision, the probation officer is caught between the judge and the offender. He has a stake in the offender's acts. He must see to it, sometimes anxiously, that the offender behaves, and he will be tempted to use further leniency during the period of probation in order to protect himself and his recommendation. Moreover, depending upon the emotional makeup of the offender, the probation officer may find himself in the curious position of condoning and covering up certain boderline antisocial acts until the offender, in further testing of the limits, commits a too flagrant abuse of probation that even this probation officer cannot tolerate. As a consequence, the new recommendation to the court may, in retaliation, be severe because of the frustration of the probation officer. The new decision may be more restrictive and punitive than it might have been in the first place if the judge had had all the facts straightforwardly presented.

Let us consider still another situation. Suppose the offender for one reason or another, perhaps because of his defiant attitude, irritated the investigating officer to the point where he is uncomfortable and, as a consequence, does not want the offender as a probationer. Instead of frankly explaining his feelings, he may try to escape this particular job of supervision by formulating his recommendation in such a way as to lead the judge to make a severe decision. If the judge rules otherwise and the offender becomes a probationer, the position of the probation officer becomes equally untenable. When challenged by the offender, who accuses him of retaliation, he cannot honestly say that his attitude is an objective one. The offender becomes more hostile, the officer more severe. Soon a flagrant, rebellious antisocial act occurs, and the probation officer has proved his point so that the judge, too, agrees that a harsher decision is necessary.

I cannot refrain from enlarging on one of the misconceptions that has resulted from the rapid development of new insights in the probation field. It is not by accident that the most skilled interpersonal workers take such a long time to produce results. The disappointing thing is that the great amount of new knowledge we acquire seems to yield much smaller dividends in the way of results than we would like. In other words, emotional growth is slow growth, lagging far behind concepts, correct as they may be. Our own intellectual awareness of new concepts far outstrips our qualitative change—the change that makes us more confident, more content, more creative, and more responsible. If we can assess this in ourselves, we can appreciate how much we may expect in the way of changes in the probationer and parolee. Because of increased knowledge we may have been led to expect faster and better results; this expectation is not valid, however, nor can we promise faster and better results to the legal authority. We deal with some of the most difficult and threatening individuals in the community, and since they are still subject to the same influences that helped make them as they are, this negates to a large extent what new experiences we have to offer. We still must depend on what we are and what we have solidly integrated along the way. In evaluating offenders for prognostic purposes, a convenient approach might be to divide them into two groups. One group would include those who commit serious antisocial acts occasionally, or "acutely," and a second group would include those who are chronic violators of the law. In the acute cases, if we deal with acute anxieties, we may eliminate the symptoms and consequently enable the individuals to live in society. With the chronic offenders, it may only be possible to nibble away slowly at anxieties as they become evident, hoping to do enough with the time and the skills we have available, within the limits of tolerance of ourselves and of the community, to make whatever inroads we can into the chronic patterns. If our immediate goal is complete rehabilitation, as measured by acceptable social behavior at all times, we may be expecting more than is reasonable and may, therefore, be doomed to failure at the start. Unless the recommendations to the court take these factors into consideration—not only what we can do, but also what we cannot be realistically expected to accomplish, despite our growing knowledge—we are misleading the court about predictable results because we are misleading ourselves. In this work, we must be prepared to fail before we can hope to succeed.

Let us discuss terms of probation that would logically follow a discussion of recommendations. If a man has failed to provide for his family or has committed a theft, are we prepared to supervise other aspects of his behavior besides that concerned with his transgression? If he frequents a bar and thus violates a condition of probation, shall we bring him before the court or shall we permit the violation of this limit? If so, what will be the effect? Are our conditions of probation and parole flexible enough? Can they be changed, and if so, how? There are other questions. Why has the expression, "I'm going to violate him," come into use by enforcement officers? Who violates the terms of probation, the offender or the officer? What about competitiveness between colleagues in the same agency? What about interagency strife? How do we work with a school that sends us a truant as a punitive gesture and then accuses the probation department of being punitive? How do we manage with sex offenders? What is prevention?

The word rapport deserves a little attention. To many, it means "being liked." But stressing limits to the offender, even if done with the best of skill, may mobilize his anger, hostility, and resentment. The relief, if limits are exercised properly, may be recognized only later. It is the lot of the person in authority to be the scapegoat for much of the psychopathology in the subordinate, and even the most skilled probation officer will be hated at times. The offender may make it seem that in merely reminding him of the terms of probation and parole, to which he has agreed at the start, the officer is doing him the greatest injustice. He will make a fuss and become accusatory, detecting and exploiting any uncertainties in the mind of the officer. He will use borderline infractions of the

148

limits in order to prove him unfair. Rapport, in the sense of being liked, appears nonexistent at these moments; but the officer may find it comforting to believe, as I do, that hostility and respect can be two sides of the same coin—that one does not bother to hate those to whom one is indifferent and that by enduring the hate without fear and counterhostility the officer will sooner or later evoke the "toward" movement that hostility desperately tries to conceal.

THE DELINQUENT AND HIS FAMILY

My final topic concerns work with children. Why is it that when we note a succession of children from the same family coming to the attention of a juvenile court—when we can predict that if Johnny, age twelve, has been made a ward of the court, Jimmy, age ten, will probably be along in a couple of years, and Bob, age eight, is on the way—why is it that we concentrate on each of the children as they come along and pay so little attention to helping the parents? Aside from what we may do for the children through helping the parents, thus adding a preventive aspect to our work, are not the parents often desperately seeking help for themselves, though indirectly?

Probation and parole work are developing, and have accomplished much on the firing line. The officer is still under pressure from many directions—the multidivisional legal structure, the articulate portion of the citizenry, some of the most serious community problems, and, not the least, the demands he makes of himself. That the work has progressed and that the outlook is optimistic is heartening. I am proud to have had some share in it.

PSYCHIATRY AND THE JUVENILE COURT:
PATTERNS OF COLLABORATION
AND THE USE OF COMPULSORY PSYCHOTHERAPY*

A. J. Gianascol

Historically, society's treatment of its younger members has
been marred by infanticide, child abandonment, and the exploitation
of child labor. Isolated humanitarian landmarks are largely the
work of charitable groups, such as the hospitals established in the
Middle Ages for foundling children and St. Vincent de Paul's efforts
on behalf of foundlings in France in the early seventeenth century.

The last decades of the eighteenth century saw the American and
French revolutions, the beginning of the Industrial Revolution, and
the revolutionary changes in psychiatric treatment initiated by
P. Pinel, of France. Rousseau, in his novels, presaged the changes
in psychology and education which would foster the development of
the child's spontaneity, curiosity, and innate abilities. The ferment
of these ideas resulted in educational play techniques which encouraged children's active exploration of their sensory environment and
development of their individual abilities. These techniques were put
into practice in the kindergarten founded by Froebel in the early
nineteenth century.

Psychiatric studies of children were initiated by Jean M. G. Itard,
a colleague of Pinel, in his classic studies of the mentally defective
"wolf-boy." Edouart Seguin went on to develop techniques for training mentally defective children, a field in which pessimism had pre-
vailed until then. In the mid-nineteenth century he came to the
United States and did much to improve institutions and training methods for the mentally defective. In 1876 he became the first president
of what is now the American Association for Mental Deficiency.

---

*Reprinted with permission from "Delinquency, the Juvenile Court,
and Child Psychiatry," California Youth Authority Quarterly, 15:24-
29, (Winter) 1962.

About the time of Pinel, Malthus published anonymously his "Essay on Population," in which he described man's basic needs to eat and procreate, an essay that later suggested to Wallace and Darwin their theories of evolution. A century thereafter, Freud began to elaborate his theory of the role of sexuality in the neuroses.

Darwin's revolutionary theory of evolution, The Origin of Species by Means of Natural Selection, published in 1859, emphasized the survival value of individual variations for the species. Thus, the natural selection, inheritance, and development of variations became a focus of interest, and Darwin's studies gave impetus to the comparative approach in biology and psychology. Darwin recorded the development of his infant son as part of his studies for his Expression of the Emotions in Animals and Man (3).

Psychology emerged as a separate discipline during the late nineteenth century, claiming as its basis the development of experimental methods. Darwin's cousin, Sir Francis Galton, studied individual differences in humans, using statistical methods and genetic techniques such as studies of twins. Galton concluded that both normal and abnormal psychological traits—e.g., genius, legal acumen, or criminality—were determined by heredity. C. Lombroso's theories of the "born criminal" may be considered an extension of Galton's emphasis on the importance of heredity in determining psychological traits. Prior to Galton, only gross formboards were available for estimating intelligence. His efforts to obtain precise measurement of mental abilities facilitated Binet's development of the standardized intelligence test about the turn of the century.

During the nineteenth century the technological applications of science accelerated the Industrial Revolution. The subsequent increase in the frequency of abuse of child labor led to many social, judicial, and charitable movements. Humanitarian efforts during the early nineteenth century were primarily aimed at the child labor laws and the "houses of refuge," from which reform schools evolved. The separation of children's courts from adult criminal courts was pioneered in Massachusetts after the Civil War and was soon followed by court appointment of the first probation officer.

The first large-scale waves of immigration into the United States occurred shortly before the mid-nineteenth century as aftermaths of the potato famine in Ireland and the political turmoil in Germany. The influx was most acute in New York City, where children were abandoned in the streets. The midcentury founding of the Children's Aid Society helped these abandoned children through free foster-home placement.

This landmark was followed by numerous similar agencies, but initially foster children had little legal protection. Shortly after the

Civil War, a mission worker in New York turned to the Society for the Prevention of Cruelty to Animals for help in the case of a child who was cruelly beaten by his foster parents. Since "the child was an animal," the society and its counsel brought legal action which resulted in a year's imprisonment for the foster mother. Similar requests for aid soon overwhelmed the society's limited facilities, and in 1874 a separate group was incorporated in New York as the Society for Prevention of Cruelty to Children. Through its efforts specific laws to protect and punish wrongs to children began to be enacted, and many similar organizations were established.

By the close of the century, the efforts of groups concerned with the welfare of children were climaxed by the establishment in Chicago, in 1899, of the first juvenile court. Roscoe Pound termed it the most significant event in the administration of justice since the signing of the Magna Charta in 1215. There, for the first time, children who had violated the law were classified as delinquents, rather than criminals, by a statute entitled: "An Act to Regulate the Treatment and Control of Dependent, Neglected and Delinquent Children." The juvenile court undertook the guidance and protection of children brought to its custody, rather than the determination of guilt and punishment.

The year 1899 can also be considered a landmark in the development of psychodynamic psychiatry: Freud published what he considered to be his greatest contribution, The Interpretation of Dreams (6). Important features of Freud's theories include his description of the role of conflictual inpulses and unconscious mental mechanisms in the formation of the symptoms of emotional disturbance, and his elaboration of how much of our conscious mental activity may be determined by unconscious processes. Freud strongly emphasized the role played by experiences during infancy and childhood in the formation of both normal and abnormal personalities. Although some of his concepts may be traced back into antiquity in the writings of philosophers, theologians, and physicians, they had assumed little academic or clinical importance until their formulation by Freud.

In 1909, Freud and Jung spoke at a symposium at Clark University. Freud (5) summarized the origin and development of his theories, and Jung described how the responses of individual family members to a word association test supported the notion that the unconscious conflicts of children were derived from those of their parents. In that same year, Clifford Beers founded the National Committee for Mental Hygiene; and Dr. William Healy established the Juvenile Psychopathic Institute for a five-year study of delinquency in collaboration with the juvenile court in Cook County, Illinois.

In 1918, a gift of $38 million to the National Committee for

Mental Hygiene established the Commonwealth Fund; with its financial support the committee developed seven demonstration child-guidance clinics throughout the United States, each using a team composed of a psychiatrist, a psychologist, and a social worker.

The child-guidance clinic, which may be our most original contribution in psychiatry, evolved from the collaborative efforts by the first juvenile court and a psychiatrist. The initial hope of the National Committee for Mental Hygiene—that such collaboration would lead to an answer to the problem of delinquency—was not realized, however.

PSYCHIATRIC INSIGHTS INTO DELINQUENCY

Attempts to alleviate the mounting problem of juvenile delinquency have involved the concerted efforts of sociologists, anthropologists, economists, legislators, lawyers, judges, physicians, and allied professions. Many important studies and investigations are proceeding in these diverse fields. The all-important question of prevention has been summarized by former Governor Edmund G. Brown of California in his fourteen-point program for the prevention of delinquency (2).

The term "delinquency" is not defined by statute in California. Since in many states it has important legal implications, and since legal, socioeconomic, and more fortuitous events may determine whether behavior is termed "delinquent," such behavior may be described as "acting-out." Acting-out may be defined as the impulsive expression of feelings by overt action or behavior. Usually the term implies that the behavior is directed against authority and is specifically forbidden by society.

For example, one individual might say to another if provoked, "Drop dead!"—a relatively innocuous expression of anger. The acting out of such feelings, however, may entail assault or even murder. Since such impulsive behavior can arise in the course of any mental illness, the term acting-out has no diagnostic specificity, though it may issue from specific psychodynamic mechanisms. The mechanisms involved in the genesis of the individual delinquent child pertain equally to the adult who chronologically may be termed a criminal rather than a delinquent. The importance of heredity cannot be overlooked. Although apparently no primary genetic factors account for delinquent behavior, the influence of heredity may perhaps operate more subtly by determining the physique and the energy or activity level of the individual.

The attempt to distinguish between socioculturally determined delinquency and that which is due to psychological conflicts may not be helpful. We must turn to the psychology of the individual to answer questions why nondelinquents exist in very high delinquency areas, or delinquents exist in areas with a low delinquency rate. As Kaplan has cogently stated, "Whatever factors we may consider as important etiologically, whether constitutional, social, economic, or cultural, the influence is finally upon the mental life of the individual and his psychological structure and function. The delinquent act is finally determined by a psychological state. We must therefore discuss it in psychological terms. We must strive to make a psychodynamic formulation."

A psychodynamic formulation recognizes the importance of unconscious mental mechanisms in determining both normal and abnormal behavior. It takes into account how both conscious and unconscious determinants of conflict are, to a significant degree, the product of the individual's experience with parents or parental surrogates, particularly during infancy and childhood. Thus, modern psychodynamic concepts reiterate, refine, and elaborate the age-old recognition of the importance of family life in forming the child's character and personality.

The interplay between unconscious and conscious mental processes may lead to a conflict between opposing impulses. Such a conflict in turn leads to anxiety, an extremely uncomfortable disruptive state, which mobilizes various psychological defenses against the conflicting impulses. These defenses include sublimation, rationalization, and many others. Usually they do not cause discomfort to an individual, but when they fail to function adequately, symptoms such as fears, morbid preoccupations, compulsions, and depression emerge. These symptoms may represent a secondary compromise solution to the conflict; if they produce conscious distress the individual may be led to consult a physician.

Briefly, then, conflicts arising in part from unconscious impulses may lead to anxiety, which in turn may lead to defense mechanisms. Finally, if defenses fail to function, various symptoms of mental disorder emerge, often leading the individual to seek medical help.

By contrast, the person who acts out his impulses may not experience the internal discomfort of anxiety or other symptoms and may not feel in need of medical help. Indeed, these persons initially may come to the attention of the court rather than the psychiatrist, and often may be described as unmotivated for seeking help. Their psychological disturbances distress others more frequently than themselves.

Early Investigations in Delinquency

Many of the historic insights contributed by Healy and Bronner, the Gluecks, and August Aichhorn are included in Searchlights on

Delinquency (4)—a volume dedicated to Aichhorn on his seventieth birthday. The various approaches to delinquency are represented in the encyclopedic compendium edited by Sheldon Glueck, The Problem of Delinquency (8).

Early investigators, such as Healy, considered broken homes, mental disorder, feeblemindedness and similar factors as contributory to the development of delinquency; and they also noted an occasional similarity between the pattern of a parent's crime and that of the child (e.g., both committed acts of aggression). These generalities now seem glib, but they served as signposts for future research.

No psychological sophistication is needed to understand the influence of a parent who asks his child to lie about his age to qualify for "no fare," or to keep an eye out the rear window for the patrol car as he exceeds the speed limit. How familiar to parents is the response of children who, when reprimanded, say, "But after all, you do the same thing. Why can't I?" Similarly, when a child is expelled from school for smoking, his parent may seem to accept the rule in a conference with the child and teacher, only to chide the child afterward, saying, "I don't care if you smoke, but you ought to know enough not to get caught!"

The wisdom of observations such as "Like father, like son" is evident. It does not seem too farfetched to consider that the child acquires his attitudes and behavior in the same way that he learns his speech—from his parents. Just as a qualified linguist can often tell by studying the child's speech where in the United States each parent had spent a considerable time, so the child psychiatrist can often predict the parents' personalities by studying the child. These gross mechanisms, whose prevalence may be obscured by the conscious denial of such attitudes by the parents, do not entirely account for the development of acting-out behavior in children. We must look further.

Freud suggested one explanation of acting-out behavior in a theory titled "Criminality from a Sense of Guilt" (7). He proposed that criminal acts are attempts by an individual to provide a realistic basis for unconscious guilt feelings, which he considered to originate from the child's oedipal feelings towards his parents. Punishment for the transgression further served to satisfy these guilt feelings. The acting-out thus seemed to provide a rational basis to which the guilt could be displaced, while the punishment served to mitigate the guilt. Freud's theory was elaborated by Alexander (1). While such guilt mechanisms may have relevance, particularly in those delinquents whose behavior seems to invite or insure detection, the hypothesis does not explain why the individual selects a particular one of many available modes for punishing himself. For example, gambling, losing a job, or "accidental" injury may all serve the same purpose.

In my experience, some instances of acting-out behavior by a delinquent represent his plea for external controls, as he becomes aware that his own internal control over his impulses may be inadequate. He may openly express his relief at apprehension, so that he cannot commit more serious crimes. In fact, some individuals who request custodial care to prevent their carrying out a serious crime—for example, murder—may indeed carry out the feared impulse if they are not detained, or may do so later when they are released.

The Parents' Part

The next advance into the dynamics of delinquency was anticipated at the Institute of Juvenile Research in Chicago by Szurek in 1942 (11) and developed in later reports with his coworkers (12). It stemmed from their development of a new treatment technique, the collaborative therapy of children and their parents. This method included the treatment of the child by a child psychiatrist and the treatment of one or both parents by the same or another child psychiatrist.

The technique enabled the therapists to scrutinize closely the psychological mechanisms at play within the family and within each individual, particularly during the early stages of the development of acting-out behavior in the child. During the course of treatment, the more subtle subconscious and unconscious determinants of behavior began to be understood, as well as the complexities of the family interaction, particularly as it impinged on the child.

In the children they studied, Johnson and Szurek (12) found defects in the conscience which they termed "superego lacunae." These defects were usually limited to an inability to control one or two specific impulses such as lying or stealing. In addition, one or both parents were found to manifest similar defects. Thus the child learned his lack of control specifically from the parents.

These correlations between the personality defects in the parents and the child were more subtle than the grosser correlations described by earlier workers. Johnson and Szurek traced how a child's acting out at times was unconsciously fostered and sanctioned by one or both parents, who thereby achieved vicarious satisfaction of their own antisocial impulses through the child's behavior. By vacillation and innuendo in their attitudes and by permissiveness or inconsistency toward the child's behavior the parents encouraged his acting-out. These parents have difficulty in clearly defining limits, either for themselves or their children, and their standards vacillate or deviate from those of society.

An example is illustrated by the father of a child referred for evaluation because of serious fire setting. Although the parent gave lip service to the antisocial nature of his child's act, he uneasily sanctioned it, stating, "There's nothing wrong with that. I used to set fires myself."

Somewhat more subtle were the mechanisms involved in an adolescent's thefts. His behavior formed part of a pattern that led up to the juvenile court hearing at which psychiatric treatment was made a condition of probation. The parents were held responsible for the boy's hospital expenses, and an equitable fee was set. The father, though financially able, persistently refused to pay it, and legal action was necessary to obtain payment. Though the father verbally condemned his son's behavior, he himself behaved in a somewhat similar way.

How the more unconscious forbidden impulses of the parent may vicariously be satisfied through the child is demonstrated by the teenager's parent or parents who repeatedly admonish the child about sexual misbehavior on dates and then wait up and question the child about the details of the evening. The questions include pressing the child for any inkling of sexual overtures, either on his part or the date's. Although initially such behavior may not have occurred to the child, eventually he catches on, particularly after his veracity is repeatedly questioned. Very often the parent's description of a child's sexual misbehavior is related with a smile, a clue to parental vicarious satisfaction.

Through these innuendos, the parents may continue to foster the child's acting out.

Parents of acting out adolescents often describe how they "looked the other way" or "winked at" certain behavior in their children which they did not consider serious. Nonverbal sanctioning of acting out behavior is not infrequent in the backgrounds of delinquent children.

But distortions may arise from these statements about the dynamics of delinquency, as then the parents ask, "Does that mean we are to blame for our child's difficulty?" To say that emotional disturbance in a child is a reflection and a result of the emotional difficulty of the parents is not meant as an accusation of parental blame. The formulation is not intended to imply any inkling in the parents that their own emotional difficulties, which were largely out of their own awareness, would cause similar or related difficulties in their child. The parents' part in bringing about the disturbance was not premeditated.

In fact, once parents become aware of how their own problems have been reflected in their children, it is often a tragic insight, with which they need help with their feelings of guilt.

PSYCHIATRIC TREATMENT OF DELINQUENTS

The discussion of the role of psychiatrists and psychiatric facilities in the treatment of juvenile delinquents must begin with the note that treatment has not been entirely encouraging; nor does psychiatric treatment necessarily hold promise for the solution of the overall problem of delinquency. Any hopes engendered about the merits of the treatment program must be limited by the small number of professional personnel available.

When a child or adolescent under age eighteen is referred to our clinic for evaluation, whether by himself, by his parents, or by any community resource, we offer to meet first with the parents or other responsible adults. If the parents feel that our resources would be useful to them in further planning for their child, we meet with the child and each parent, both together and individually over a period of several weeks. During this time we study the child with all the skills available to our medical center, including psychiatric, psychological, physical, and laboratory examinations, as well as a detailed review of the child's and parents' histories. Our goal is to understand, with the parents, the events and stresses they and the child have experienced which may be related to the child's current disturbance. From this formulation we then explore with the parents the treatment alternatives that are available within the community facilities and how they might wish to proceed.

The treatment program for the child at our institute involves the child's being seen on a regular basis for at least one interview a week; each parent is also seen for an hour of individual psychotherapy per week. The parents are thus offered the opportunity for treatment to see if a reduction in their own conflicts can thereby reduce both their own tensions and those of their child. Treatment is conducted under the supervision and direction of a child psychiatrist. The therapist may be a psychiatrist, psychologist, or psychiatric social worker, depending on the needs of the family and the availability of staff time.

A difficulty in the psychiatric treatment of delinquents is that they or their parents may not seek treatment voluntarily. Those who begin without any "community coercion" from school or courts seldom continue. Another difficulty is that in these patients and their families the tendency to act out hinders effective participation in treatment. We therefore feel it may be helpful if, when a child is before the court, compulsory psychotherapy for the child with the parents' participation is made a condition for probation. Such a liaison between the court and the therapist need not interfere with therapy.

The therapist's role in helping the patient and his parents to better understand themselves is clearly defined. The therapist is not a substitute for the probation officer. This does not mean, however, that the therapist will not communicate to the court or to the patient's parents any violations of the conditions of probation. This is made explicit to the patient and to the family.

It is always important to appreciate the conscious or unconscious attempts by the delinquent to manipulate authority figures into participation in his acting-out. Thereby he seeks to demonstrate that his acting-out is justified because "you do it, too." Even when removed from his family, the delinquent attempts, consciously or unconsciously, to provoke others into assuming the roles his parents previously had played. For example, the probation officer may be unwittingly involved in the patient's acting-out when the patient fails to keep an appointment with his psychiatrist in order to keep an impromptu appointment he has arranged with his probation officer. This continued testing by the delinquent—and sometimes by his parents, too—necessitates constant and close collaboration between the probation officer and the psychotherapist, as well as between them and others involved in the delinquent's social setting, whether community agencies or the school. Indeed the frequency and mode of acting-out by the delinquent are often a sensitive index to the efficiency of the program collaboration.

REFERENCES

1. ALEXANDER, F., & STAUB, H. The criminal, the judge, and the public. Transl. by Gregory Zilborg. New York: MacMillan, 1931.

2. BROWN, Gov. E. B. 14 points for delinquency prevention. Sacramento: California State Printing Office, 1960.

3. DARWIN, C. The expression of the emotions in man and animals. New York: Philosophical Library, 1955.

4. EISSLER, K. R. (Ed.), Searchlights on delinquency. New York: International Universities Press, 1949.

5. FREUD, S. The origin and development of psychoanalysis. Transl. by H. W. Chase. Am. J. Psychol., 21:181-218, 1910.

6. FREUD, S. The interpretation of dreams. Transl. by A. A. Brill. In A. A. Brill (Ed.), The basic writing of Sigmund Freud. New York: Random House, 1938.

7. FREUD, S. Some character-types met with in psychoanalytic work. In Collected Papers, Vol. IV. London: Hogarth Press, 1948.

8. GLUECK, S. The problem of delinquency. Boston: Houghton Mifflin, 1959.

9. JOHNSON, A., & SZUREK, S. A. The genesis of antisocial acting out in children and adults. Psychoanal. Quart., 21:323-343, 1952. (See page 13 of this volume.)

SUGGESTED ADDITIONAL READINGS

CRUTCHER, R. Child psychiatry: A history of its development. Psychiatry, 6:191-201, 1943.

DE BEAUMONT, G., & DE TOQUEVILLE, A. On the penitentiary system in the United States and its application in France. Transl. with intro., notes, and additions, by Francis Lieber. Philadelphia: Carey, Lea and Blanchard, 1833.

FAYNE, G. H. The child in human progress. New York: G. P. Putnam's Sons, 1916.

LOWREY, L. C. (Ed.) Orthopsychiatry, 1923-1948: Retrospect and prospect. New York: Amer. Orthopsychiat. Assn., 1948.

WITMER, H. Psychiatric clinics for children. New York: Commonwealth Fund, 1940.

ZIETZ, D. Child welfare: Principles and methods. New York: Wiley, 1959.

ZILBOORG, G., & HENRY, G. W. A history of medical psychology. New York: W. W. Norton, 1941.

PSYCHIATRIC COMMENT ON THE PROBLEMS
OF POLICE WORK WITH DELINQUENTS*

R. W. Brunstetter

The role of the police officer is a pivotal one in the prevention of delinquency. The function of the police is to protect life and property, and to preserve the public peace. The firm, constant exercise of this function is a vital part of work with delinquents, since it defines clearly and repeatedly the limits that the society in which they are about to become adults has set upon the behavior of its members.

There are a number of other ways in which the police officer participates in the prevention of delinquency. He can develop a personal knowledge of the teenagers in his area and, by so doing, forestall crime or minimize its consequences. He can anticipate trouble by identifying problem areas such as drive-ins and pool halls, and by working with the adults in charge to make them a less explosive situation. He can get to know the community services in his neighborhood, the job opportunities, and the recreational facilities. He can recognize the delinquent leaders and give them special attention, knowing that they can exercise influence for good as well as bad if given the opportunity.

Like the doctor or minister or lawyer, the police officer is on exhibit. Youngsters watch him, perhaps unconsciously, to see whether he's got something that they want. If he can demonstrate in his demeanor and manner of living that maturity and lawfulness are ends to be sought after, he may serve as a kind of ego model for uncertain, searching children.

When the policeman advances on a stolen car with a defiant teenager behind the wheel, he can be sure of one thing—this is no chance occurrence that is happening. It is not a scene isolated in time and unconnected with anything. The sullen teenager has taken a long, long time to get to where he is, and what he faces is a moment of

---

*Unpublished, 1968.

truth in which he has stepped clearly beyond the bounds, not just in fantasy and not in his own family where he can get away with it, but out in society and "for real." Much of his future may depend on how society and its representative, the police officer, meets him at this point.

In the writer's experience, many delinquents begin as neurotic children. For one reason or another—perhaps partly for physical reasons or because of parental problems—their infancy does not give them what infants are supposed to get: a basic, deeply in-grained sense of trust in the world and in the fact that everything is fundamentally right. They approach the developmental tasks of early childhood with insecurity and apprehension. Their histories reveal many evidences of tension at this time: head-banging, finger-sucking, tantrums, fear of separation from the mother, iso-lated play, and delayed speech. The test of school and of adjust-ment outside the sheltered home proves too much. They do not learn to read and so fall behind in school. Their already tenuous self-esteem grows less every day with each fresh failure in school and in front of their peers. They have to hide this from themselves. To get rid of tension, their behavior becomes impulsive and dis-orderly. Their parents prove unable to help them with this begin-ning shift. Although consciously furious at the child for his behavior, they unconsciously, because of their own conflicts and disappoint-ments, identify with his rebellion and hence cannot deal with it. The delinquent adaptation becomes more habitual for the child. His life is a constant round of failure and punishment, promises and tears; but the feeling of anxiety does begin to become less promi-nent in his awareness. He discovers other ways of getting things than by going to school, which becomes more and more impossible. He finds friends who feel the same way that he does. He lies, he steals a little, and he becomes a truant. His parents are furious with him, but one way or another they always give in or stop short of helping him. Authority becomes his enemy. He stalks it in many little ways, in fantasy and in real life—goading it, testing it, trying to make it give him what he wants when he wants it and with-out working for it. When he goes too far, authority angrily strikes back at him; then he feels sorry for himself and has even more reason to hate because everything is "unfair."

All this is part of the delinquent's past by the time he reaches his first contact with the official authority of society in the person of the arresting officer. This is a crisis, a point of no return. He will try to see this authority as he has seen all others in the past: rigid and punishing but also, underneath, vacillatory and weak. His behavior is an attempt to get the authority he is facing to treat him the way he expects to be treated. The officer who yields and loses his temper or finds it easier to let him off does the delinquent little good, for this only proves that his view of the world is the right one—even in the "big time." It may give him something to boast about to his friends.

It is important that the arresting officer resist the provocations of the delinquent and remain firm and, as far as is possible, fair in his exercise of his lawful functions. Such a state of mind and behavior may not be easy to achieve. Policemen are human, and they react to the stresses and tensions of the situation like anyone else. There are many problems connected with just performing the job at hand at the scene of an arrest. An investigation has to be made and a decision arrived at as to whether a crime has probably been committed. If so, another decision has to be made about arrest, another about referral to the juvenile court, and still another about detention. None of these is easy to make. Any reasonable police officer cannot help but sometimes be concerned about whether he has made the right decisions. In these days of citizen attention to police methodology, he is open to criticism from the public as well as from his superiors. Furthermore, it must inevitably happen that the teenager is big enough or drunk enough or surrounded by an ugly enough crowd that the officer feels a certain amount of physical fear within himself that he must handle.

The delinquent often goads and tests the police officer in a number of different ways: by lying, by making him feel unfair and uncertain, by provoking him to retaliate, and by being insulting, sullen, and uncooperative. The feelings this gives rise to are difficult to handle. Certain aspects of them are worthy of more detailed consideration.

Unfairness. In our times, with psychiatry in the ascendancy, it is a common assumption that unfairness to children, especially those who are disturbed, is to be avoided at any cost. Yet it is important to remember that it is the consequences of his or his parents' actions, rather than the teenager's own sometimes belligerent and self-pitying judgments, that must be attended to in deciding whether a given course of action is truly fair or unfair. Anyone who tries not to be unfair to a delinquent may soon find himself in a bewildering maze of concessions and uncertain efforts to be understanding. The delinquent may, for instance, at the moment of his arrest so present himself that the officer has real doubts as to whether he understands the situation or is being fair in making the arrest. However, he is only feeling what the delinquent's parents have felt before him many times over. Delinquents' distrust is born out of bitter experience with the broken promises and selfishness of adults, but by the time they become adolescents many delinquents have become callously adroit at exploiting the worship of fairness in our society. They whipsaw their parents with it and back them into tighter and tighter corners, demanding equal rights and privileges at every turn and allowing no hint of differential treatment or arbitrariness to go unchallenged.

But the pursuit of fairness has its limits, and other, more important things should not be sacrificed for its sake. One must be willing sometimes to run the risk of being unfair in order to be firm in the requirement that what must be done must be done. It is enough to want to be fair and to do everything possible to be so; to do more may be to lose sight of more important goals and fail to be truly helpful. Probably many more youngsters have been hurt by being allowed to get away with questionable offenses over and over again than have ever been seriously injured by the occasional unfair arrest.

Punishment. Transgression of the law invites punishment. Yet it is a curious thing that nothing does less to prevent further transgression than punishment which is retaliatory and eliminates the possibility of restitution. The lesson intended is somehow never learned. Instead, the person who is punished tends to concentrate on his hurt, his resentment, and his wishes for vengeance rather than on improvement in himself.

The behavior of a delinquent may incite anger in a police officer and an urge to punish and retaliate. If the officer follows this urge in either deed or word, he confirms the delinquent's hostile attitude toward authority. It can also prove dangerous. There can occur a kind of escalation of threatening action between officer and offender. In one instance, for example, an officer who was taunted beyond endurance finally swore at a suspect he was questioning and drew his gun. When the mother tried to intervene, she was shoved rudely aside. The suspect responded to this insult by grabbing a rifle from the wall of his room and breaking the policeman's arm with the butt. He ran out of the house into the night and crouched behind the stairs in the backyard. The policeman's partner followed him and from the top of the stairs picked him out with the beam from his flashlight. Every time he did so, the suspect aimed his rifle at the light. Finally it was necessary to shoot him. There is futility and danger in retaliation because it provokes further aggression and because it leaves people no way out without losing face.

The delinquent may exploit a reluctance to punish in the same way that he does the avoidance of unfairness. In our child-oriented society, punishment has acquired unfortunate connotations, and frequently, in attempting to avoid what may be vindictive or retaliatory in their impulses to punish, parents abandon altogether their responsibility for demonstrating clearly to their child by appropriately responsive actions the consequences of his behavior and the limits which society, and they themselves, would customarily set upon it.

In psychiatric work with parents of delinquents, for instance, there often comes a time when it is perfectly clear that the youngster is saying, in effect, "I can get away with anything I want to because you're afraid to punish me or risk hurting me or even my feelings." If the parent can be helped to respond to such circumstances with limiting behavior and with a clear statement that it is the situation his teenager has brought about, rather than his own uncontrolled feelings, that leads him to do so—that parent has made a major step forward toward the solution of his family's problems.

Emotions. It is the hallmark of the delinquent that he arouses in those who have to deal with him many feelings about which they are confused and ashamed. Ranging from anger through fear and guilt, the catalog of such emotions is almost infinitely varied and includes most of the unpleasant states of mind known to man. Many people try to hide their feelings from themselves and others. They think that there is something wrong with them for feeling that way. The fact of the matter is, however, that almost everybody does, to one degree or another. The principal danger lies not in having such feelings but in what can happen when they are repressed and denied until some final incident produces a real explosion. If the feelings of anxiety or anger can be acknowledged to oneself as well as to others, they can provide useful interpersonal information about the delinquent's behavior, and seldom will lead to difficulty or criticism. Other people are more likely to feel relieved than they are to feel critical, since they are usually struggling with the same feelings themselves.

Authority. In the final analysis, the issue for the juvenile delinquent is the issue of authority. The nature of his difficulty is clarified by the distinction Szurek has drawn between two essentially different kinds of authority (see Chapter 4). One is authoritarian—dictator-like and characterized by immaturity on the part of both persons. The relationship between them is a sado-masochistic one which contains much selfishness and depends on restrictiveness to maintain its existence. The other is authoritative, which is a more mature relationship in which the authority is genuinely interested in helping the person under him to develop so that he can ultimately achieve equal status.

A delinquent has gotten into trouble all of his life because of impulses he wants gratified immediately. His parents are authoritarian and immature. They deny him gratification because it conflicts with their own pleasures, or they allow themselves to be bullied and in so doing indulge him and, vicariously, themselves. More often than not they vacillate between these two extremes. The delinquent needs an authoritative relationship with someone who has a genuine interest in his welfare and can firmly and without retaliation, even in the face of anger, oppose the impulse toward wrongdoing without ceasing to be supportive and accepting of the teenager himself. The authoritative person knows, for instance, that conflicted sexual and aggressive impulses can be mastered because he himself has mastered them in the course of reaching maturity. He knows that true gratification is not something to be obtained immediately, but that all things worthwhile—including respect, love, and station in life—require time and effort to achieve them. Knowing this, he teaches by example the value and meaning of patience.

A delinquent has not had the benefit of this kind of relationship with his parents. Police officers who have frequent dealings with parents of delinquents often find them as baffling and infuriating as their teenagers. For a long time, in fact, there has been a school of thought in connection with delinquency which has insisted that the way to stop it is to punish parents for the transgressions of their children, thus wringing from them a measure of the responsibility they often seem unwilling by themselves to assume. Laws like this have been passed in some communities but, when enforced, have failed to be helpful. This is understandable for many reasons, not the least of which is that it puts still another club in the hands of a mixed-up teenager who already is adept at controlling and punishing his family with his behavior. The truth is that most detailed psychiatric investigations have shown that the parents of delinquent children are themselves involved in serious neurotic difficulties and that their relationships with their children are almost totally beyond their control by a simple act of will. They are helped by punitiveness even less than their children. The delinquent's parents may demonstrate to the arresting officer the same kinds of behavior that the teenager has at his command. They may be threatening and abusive. Many of them want to protect their boy or girl from contact with the law, and they are willing to use influence or bully or bribe to do so. Others are so angry that they just want to get rid of their youngster.

There is a temptation to use parents as a convenient scapegoat and to take out on them the anger which is felt toward the delinquent but denied expression. Nevertheless, it is as important with the parents as with the teenager to be understanding and non-retaliative, but firm in seeing to it that what needs to be done at the moment for their good and for society's protection is done promptly and thoroughly.

The delinquent is generally a deeply conflicted person who has learned to control his disorder by evading responsibility, by satisfying his impulses immediately, and by dominating and exploiting those around him with his misbehavior. He comes from a troubled family. His parents have the same kinds of problems but they are more buried and often come to light only around their youngster. The delinquent needs a great deal of understanding but understanding is not the same thing as indulgence. In fact, the very thing that needs to be understood most about him is his need for firm limits and controls. The most helpful thing that a police officer can do in dealing with a juvenile delinquent is to be a good police officer. Effective law enforcement is the beginning of prevention and treatment.

REFERENCES

1. SZUREK, S. A. Emotional factors in the use of authority. In Public health is people. New York: Commonwealth Fund, 1950. (See page 48 of this volume.)

THE ROLE OF THE PSYCHIATRIST
IN A PROBATION AGENCY*

Samuel Susselman

The work of a probation agency can be enhanced by the aid of a psychiatrist. The addition of a psychiatrist to the staff means ideally the acquisition of a participant worker who can share with others what he knows while learning from them what they know. How he functions depends upon the needs and sophistication of the agency and of the psychiatrist. These determine whether his activities are confined to diagnostic interviews or extended to other matters. For example, should he teach psychodynamics? Should he advise on management or disposition of cases? Should he have anything to do with the schools and the collaborating social agencies? How much should he be expected to offer in the way of diagnosis or advice to the judge, the referee, the probation officer, the detention personnel? All these are questions to be worked out collaboratively. Other questions that arise are related to the psychiatrist's training and experience. For example, is the psychiatrist psychoanalytically oriented? Has he had training in child psychiatry, in work with social agencies? The aim is to integrate the activities of the psychiatrist with those of the agency in order to attain their mutual goal, which is more effective functioning of the agency. It is my purpose here to present a worker-oriented (1) philosophy of psychiatric consultation that can, potentially, help to resolve many agency problems and that may contribute to the growth and development of the agency.

It will be useful first to discuss a fundamental concept, that of the relationship of emotional conflict to authority. (See also Chapter 4 of this volume.) At birth an infant is endowed with biological and emotional impulses that must be at least partially satisfied if he is to survive. The parents are the agents through whom the

---

*Reprinted with permission from <u>Focus</u>, 29(3):33, 1950. (Copyright, the National Council on Crime and Delinquency.)

168

child is educated to take his place, first in the home and later in society. In the process of acculturation certain of his impulses will be interfered with, and he will seek substitute ways of expression. Frustrated, he will try to circumvent interfering obstacles. He may react with a revengeful attack upon the obstacle, in some instances the parents. His subjective feelings are those of rage and anger, feelings that may not be readily expressed for fear of the consequences. He may, therefore, find it more feasible to suppress overt actions and feelings by retiring from what have become to him danger-laden attempts at expression. This leaves him with pent-up emotion that makes him uncomfortable and unhappy. When he is in such a state we say he is anxious, meaning that he is in conflict. Any behavioral manifestations now are distortions of the original impulse; we see the evasive child, the rebellious child, or the inhibited, neurotic child.

This is the child's first encounter with authority. The manner in which the parent intervenes in the face of these unacceptable impulses and deals with the resultant rage contributes to the future personality traits of the child. If the parent is sufficiently unanxious, the problem is minimal. He will genuinely wish to teach the child to gain satisfactions in ways that are least destructive to himself and his environment. The parent will guide the child so that eventually he will become relatively happy and secure in society. This parent will act unambivalently and clearly.

ANXIETY AND AUTHORITY RELATIONS

The insecure parent, well-intentioned but unsure of himself and therefore more vulnerable, will react with more than his usual uncertainty when the demands of the child threaten him in some way. This indicates a struggle going on within him similar to that within the child. The demands of the child increase this conflict, causing the insecure parent more uneasiness and anxiety. Not only does this anxiety obscure the issue between parent and child, but it often leads to irrational behavior by the parent. He now has to deal with his own feelings in a troublesome area, something he has never done quite adequately.

In these circumstances, he will be unable to help the child as effectively as can the less anxious parent. He may vacillate about preventing his child from doing something he himself is tempted to do, almost telling the child to seek gratification as best he can. The weak "no" uttered by the parent, in comparison to a firm "no," is almost tantamount to "yes." This is probably why the parent is often heard to say, "I just don't know why my son does just the opposite of what I tell him to do." On the other hand, if the parent, driven by his own internal conflicts and consequent anxieties, attempts to be really firm, he tends to be too strict. His firmness becomes unduly suppressive; it is rigid and is not based on his good judgment.

The child may react with defiance. As a consequence, he may become distrustful of all authority, ready to react defensively and often self-destructively, as he did to the ambivalently expressed authority of his parents. He grows apart from his group, his aggressiveness estranges him from his fellow man and his fellow man from him. As he grows, he may interpret even judicious authority as evil, for he has known no other kind. Rebelliously, he may do just the opposite of what he is told. Less easily recognized is the problem of the child who becomes unduly submissive, whose neurotic difficulties are not apparent early in life but whose disability is often more marked when it is discovered. Sometimes physical complaints or habit disturbances are the evidence of the internal struggle.

Reduction of Anxiety

During psychiatric training many of us learn for the first time about those occasions on which we become involved in emotional conflicts of our own and behave in non-therapeutic ways. At these times our assumed omnipotence may be a cloak covering underlying insecurity; we may engage in sibling rivalry with our colleagues for the approbation of our supervisors; we may tend to ingratiate ourselves with our patients in our need to be liked; and we may be hostile to some patients and vacillating with others. Just as in the parent-child relationship, these feelings are directed not only toward our patients, but also toward our associates. We react with anxieties that we try to mask by actions resembling those of the anxious parent described above. Such behavior may tend to perpetuate the neurosis of the patient instead of helping him. We may even come to an impasse in treatment. When, in our supervisory hours or in talks with friendly and aware colleagues, we discover and understand our own problems we feel relieved. We experience a resolution of conflict and a freedom from anxiety that allows us to proceed again with the patient with a new objectivity, for we are no longer as emotionally involved. Even when these discussions fail to reveal any specific problem, relief may occur. I am sure that you have in times of stress talked to a friend who is calm and unanxious, and from whom you return with a feeling of objectivity and a reassurance that things will turn out well. At least you feel better able to cope with your problems. This experience is so common that psychotherapy is sometimes said to be a process in which the less anxious one helps the more anxious one to become less anxious.

The efficacy of this process is revealed in a situation familiar to any intake worker, whether she serves in a social agency, a psychiatric clinic, or a juvenile court. A frantic mother in search of help telephones the intake worker at a psychiatric clinic. Her Johnny has been having temper tantrums and has been teasing his little sister to such a degree that the home is upset and the mother is at her wit's end. She's tried everything; Johnny has been talked to, punished, and rewarded, but with no improvement. She has to have an appointment immediately. The social worker hears the mother out and discusses with her the development of the problem, without becoming involved in the mother's anxiety. Often this results in a reduction in the pressure the mother feels, and she may agree to wait for the first appointment hour that can be offered, sometimes several days away. At the designated time the mother appears. Her opening statement is often, "I don't know whether or not I should be here. A funny thing happened. Since I talked with you on the phone, Johnny has been swell. He's hardly been any trouble at all."

Again, Mary, a schizophrenic twelve-year-old patient, was as physically mature as an eighteen-year-old. One day she suddenly and violently beat a six-year-old girl who had been annoying her. Two days later, Mary again became violent, and had to be forcibly locked in isolation on an adult ward. Nurses and attendants felt that something had to be done. A careful review of the events leading up to the violent outbreak was undertaken. Bit by bit, the story emerged. Due to staff shortages, only one nurse was in attendance on the children's ward that night. She had been apprehensive about Mary, who, shortly after the nurse came on duty, began to run up and down the dormitory, patently excited. The nurse had said, "Mary, if you don't stop that, I'll have to put you in a room by yourself." Mary agreed. They went to a vacant room, but there was no bed. The nurse turned to Mary and said, "You'll have to help me push your bed into this room." The girl cooperated. After the door was shut, they peered at each other for a moment through the glass and then the nurse impulsively and fearfully locked the door. Immediately Mary exploded. She broke the tumbler and mirror in the toilet and screamed. Help was summoned, and she was forcibly placed on the adult ward.

In reviewing the situation, it seemed clear that when the nurse in her professional role somehow dealt with her own anxiety, Mary, bigger and stronger than she, complied sufficiently to go into the room and even helped push in the bed. It also seemed that at the moment when Mary and the nurse were viewing each other through the glass, the nurse had a return surge of anxiety and locked the door. The outbreak was thereby precipitated. Recognizing how frightening it was to the nurse to be alone on the ward with Mary and the other children, the supervisor made help easily available, should Mary again become threatening. Reassured by this, the nurse agreed to return to the ward that night alone, and in the year since then, Mary has had no violent episodes. The patient inquiry by the psychiatrist; the appreciation of the uneasiness of the frightened nurse, who felt her responsibility keenly and blamed herself for her failure to meet a trying situation; the setting of the stage so the nurse could, without embarrassment, verbalize her feelings in the presence of others—all contributed to a reduction of anxiety in the nurse and the evolving of a plan of operation which she found acceptable. She also learned that when she could recognize and deal with her own anxiety, she could be more helpful.

Consultation as Anxiety Reduction

Let us consider how this important insight, the reduction of anxiety, can be utilized in psychiatric consultive work in a probation agency. That same anxiety-reducing process which appears so helpful to the psychiatrist, the social worker, the parent, and the nurse may also be helpful to the probation officer who, in his work, has become entangled in his own conflicts. The probation officer, within the limits of his time and ability, handles without undue difficulty the majority of the cases to which he is assigned. How does it happen that one particular client causes him such concern that he refers the case to the psychiatrist? Perhaps the following summaries will suggest some answers.

Ann had been known to the juvenile court as a destitute child when she was nine years old. The family background was complicated. The mother's numerous marital and extramarital relationships produced five children by several men. At age fifteen Ann, the second child, was placed in a boarding school, where she was reported to be sulky, untruthful, and uninterested in the usual activities. At sixteen she complained about being discriminated against. On a visit home she became ill with an upset stomach and nervous headaches. Within two days she had found her way back to the school and was discovered in the nursery in a dazed condition; her sleeves were torn to the shoulder, and her face was grimy as though someone had placed his hand over her mouth. She said she wanted to go home again and stay home; and when the request was not granted, she took twenty pills in a suicide attempt. It was learned from her mother that Ann had threatened suicide several times. Three months later the school returned her to the juvenile court because Ann claimed to see visions of God, and was upset when no one else could see these apparitions.

She was committed to a state hospital, ran away five months later, and was returned. At that time, Ann was bored with other girls, and used too much profane language. Her behavior was bizarre, and she preferred a deteriorated adult ward to the children's unit. The following spring, when she was considered ready for discharge, one of the social work agencies stated: "It would appear that there is no institution or foster home prepared to cope with the problems presented by Ann at this time, nor with the problems we anticipate. We regret we cannot accept Ann's placement."

About a year after entering the hospital, she was returned to her home, where she adjusted poorly. A foster home with friends of the family was next tried by her mother. There she became hysterical one day and told the family that she had been at the state hospital. The foster mother became upset at the idea of harboring an insane person, especially since Ann kept repeating, "My sister says I'm crazy, maybe I am crazy." Ann, now seventeen and indeed a problem, was returned to detention with no plan in sight.

The probation officer did everything possible to make Ann happy. She took her shopping one day for clothes, but after her first enthusiasm Ann lost interest and finally selected clothes in no way suitable. On the detention floor, she had difficulty in adjusting to the other girls, feeling apart from the group.

At this time, she was referred to me for a psychiatric interview. Her mother was interviewed as well, and despite her history of being uncooperative, she gave the impression that she herself might consider psychotherapy. Soon a foster home for Ann was found with a woman ready to accept the challenge Ann represented; but this too failed, and Ann was again returned to the detention floor. She made continued demands upon her probation officer, sent her on trips to get phonograph records, asked for money and clothes, and was never satisfied.

At this point the probation officer, who was uncertain what to do next, requested a conference. We had become well enough acquainted so that she could express her feelings freely. As we carefully examined everything she said, we discovered her feelings of hopelessness and futility about Ann, together with her need to succeed with this very disturbed girl, who was such a drain on her time and her emotions. The consultation helped her recognize how difficult it had always been for anyone to succeed with Ann, who had defeated everyone who had made any attempt to help her. She realized anew, and perhaps for the first time in this case, that failure was no disgrace. When she felt somewhat more at ease, it was suggested that if she felt ready, she might tell Ann that although she would be glad to spend time with her, pressure of other work made this difficult; further, that she would be glad to supply Ann with things and to do errands for her, but only within the limits of the time available. Surprisingly enough, Ann reacted favorably to this change and in a short time stopped making demands. Repeated unambivalent contact with the probation officer, who was now dealing with Ann more easily, had the same quieting effect. Soon one of the recreation workers became interested in Ann, who began to adjust to other girls.

Ann later was transferred to a home for girls, where she continued her good adjustment. Meanwhile, the mother was in frequent communication with the probation officer, who was able also to deal adequately with her, and Ann was eventually returned to her home. At times of stress the mother called the probation officer, and each time was helped to cope with her daughter. Ten months later, Ann was making at least as good an adjustment as she ever had. The mother had moved closer to obtaining psychotherapy for herself and for Ann, and was scheduled for an early appointment.

As a result of the one conference described above, the problem was clarified with the probation officer so that she could proceed. Her ability to deal with this difficult case had existed at the time of the conference, but was obscured by her emotional involvement. Helping her to view the situation objectively permitted her to use these abilities constructively.

In another case, a probation officer was in a quandary about a difficult situation. Two children had been taken into court custody when their mother became psychotically depressed and was committed to a state hospital, and they were referred by the court to a collaborating agency for foster-home placement. The father repeatedly interfered with the activities of this agency and criticized its procedures. He became so upset at times that the agency worker felt that the father too required committment to a mental hospital. When the mother was returned to the home, improved but requiring periodic visits to the hospital, the father insisted that the children be returned. The agency worker complied. However, she told the probation officer that home was a poor place for the children and that steps should be taken to commit the father to a state hospital. The probation officer visited the home and talked with the parents, but did not agree that the children should be removed. He spoke also with the mother's sister, a reliable informant, who reported that things were going well in the home. The mother had never seemed better. The probation officer could not, of course, take action.

My discussion with the probation officer brought out what had been troubling him: if the mother again became psychotic or if the father became mentally ill, he would once more need the cooperation of the agency personnel in returning the children to foster-home care. Would they help out when he had failed to carry out their recommendation? He was asked if he might feel able to telephone the agency worker and explain his dilemma. He might also admit the possibility that this chaotic home would soon crumble, and if so, he would again need their help; though he did not want to place himself in a position where the agency might refuse to be of service, he still would very much like to have the children remain with their parents. When he finally telephoned, being then more at ease with himself and less defensive (after all, the agency worker could very well be correct in her dire predictions), she agreed to his plans.

For the past year, the situation in this home has been stable. The father, no longer disturbed by the hostile attitude that he evoked in the agency, now deals with an accepting probation officer. His paranoid tendencies have not been apparent, and he has even invited the probation officer to join a fraternal organization. The mother's good adjustment has continued.

A few words about the general conduct of these conferences may be helpful. If other workers are present, they also can see pertinent issues and can be helpful in resolving them. Other members of the group can gain important insights into their own problems from a case under discussion. Many of the questions raised by one individual turn out to be of interest to others. One must be on guard, however, to recognize and protect a sensitive individual from interpersonal hostility, however veiled, that may appear in such group meetings. Colleagues may, on the other hand, be marvelously sensitive to the anxieties of others and be able to help when the consultant has been obtuse. Sometimes one must end a conference without reaching a conclusion, and then later meet alone with the individual most involved. If the material is presented extemporaneously without use of charts or prepared papers, it is often easier to detect the central problem, for, as in free association, the core of the difficulty is often uppermost.

PROBLEMS IN CONSULTATION

I do not want to leave the impression that I, as a psychiatric consultant, have been uniformly successful in dealing with problems that arouse anxiety in workers. Some of the things over which I may stumble are my own blind spots and the limitations of my particular professional experience. While certain time-proved methods seem to be successful for experienced workers,

other workers demand omnipotent advice. "Tell me what to do,"
is their cry, as if the psychiatrist alone knows the answer that the
worker often carries within himself. Others may attempt to seduce
the psychiatrist into taking sides against a worker, a supervisor,
or a referee who has proved difficult. Without conscious intent
they may say, "Well, the psychiatrist says . . ." A psychiatric
examination may be used as a source of information when the probation officer is pressed for time and is too busy to conduct a
social investigation before the hearing.

Finally, regardless of the awareness of either the worker or
the psychiatrist, their efforts can be completely obstructed by
another person at any level. What is the good of therapeutic interviews with a child if no one deals with the problems of the detention attendant, and the child suffers as a consequence? What is the
good of elaborate conferences if the judge or the referee, who has
not participated in the discussion, comes to a decidedly contrary
conclusion because he has not been fully informed? If collaboration among all the skilled professionals, of which the psychiatrist
is but one, has any merit, it must be all-inclusive to be effective.
I should like to see social workers, psychologists, psychiatrists,
probation workers, school personnel, judges, referees, all those
involved in a case, sit down together before adjudication to think
out the problem presented by that case. Meanwhile, an approach
to worker-oriented psychiatric consultation may make its contribution by helping to free knowledge and skills for more efficient
work.

To summarize, psychiatric consultation can be useful to a probation agency when it is effectively integrated into the function of
the agency and when the psychiatrist utilizes his skills primarily
to help to reduce tensions. These skills include, among others,
close listening, careful inquiry, attention to the sequence of events,
discernment of alternatives, and the ascertainment of formulated
agency policies and the limits of a worker's time and tolerance
when they seem blurred. In addition, the psychiatrist, especially
if he has been trained to work with children and their families,
brings explicit information about how the child can be helped by
helping those significant individuals who interact with him, the
professional worker as well as the parent. It goes withot saying
that the psychiatrist must pay careful attention to his own involvements in order to take corrective steps for himself.

REFERENCES

1. COLEMAN, J. U. Psychiatric consultation in case work agencies. Am. J. Orthopsychiat., 17(3), 1947.

2. SZUREK, S. A. Emotional factors in the use of authority. In Public health is people. New York: Commonwealth Fund, 1950. (See page 48 of this volume.)

SECTION FIVE

MENTAL HEALTH CONSULTATION TO COMMUNITY AGENCIES

INTRODUCTION

Mental health consultation has become one of the specific skills to be taught in community psychiatry. A body of knowledge, techniques, and dynamic methodology has slowly evolved, which can now be communicated to trainees in child psychiatry as well as trainees and workers in all the mental health professions. The following papers describe some aspects of the consultative process and a specific methodology for teaching and learning.

MENTAL HEALTH CONSULTATION
WITH A JUVENILE PROBATION DEPARTMENT*

I. N. Berlin

Juvenile probation officers are faced with rather specific problems which stem from the authoritative nature of their work. They find that, in working with angry, defiant delinquents, sexually misbehaving young people, and their often indifferent and disturbed parents, the fears, anxieties, and hostilities common to all human beings are highlighted and aggravated. They find, too, that the problems these young people present impinge upon the specific experiences of the workers' own past.

Mental health consultation may be helpful in reducing the tensions of the officers by helping them function more effectively as they begin to understand how to deal differently with the job's specific problems and anxieties. They then can more accurately assess the effectiveness of their work, their goals, and how they might begin to achieve these goals.

My services as mental health consultant with a juvenile probation department in central California began as a result of a community interagency agreement to hire a psychiatrist as consultant to several child-serving agencies. The intent was to help the school, probation, health, and welfare departments increase their effectiveness in dealing with their clients, so that when a community mental health clinic was opened it would not be overwhelmed by referrals. Only those persons with the most severe and urgent problems would be referred to the clinic.

Although I was hired as part of a package deal, the contracting agencies were not very clear as to what real help I could offer and what methods I would use in my work. The chief probation officer

*Reprinted with permission from Crime and Delinquency, January, 1964, 10:67-73.

was caught in a dilemma which he later described as follows: he had to endorse a community-sponsored service and yet had no conviction about his agency's need for it and no understanding of how it could be helpful. Even after some time, his feelings about having a psychiatrist in his agency were ambivalent. For the first several months, therefore, my monthly consultation meetings were taken up with lectures to the staff about child development and parent-child relationships, and with discussions of the diagnostic categories of mental illness in children and adults. In the lectures I presented several case histories and experiences from my work with adolescent delinquents and their parents, highlighting the difficulties I had encountered. I attempted also to speculate about the factors involved in several failures. I hoped these examples would give the officers a feeling that I might be able to understand their problems.

AGENCY-SPECIFIC PROBLEMS

After each lecture period, I was given an office in which to consult with any of the probation officers who had special problems. The chief probation officer did not draw up a schedule of appointments or specifically encourage his supervisors to ask their workers to bring special matters to me for consultation. For many weeks I sat alone in the office, receiving an occasional visit from a curious probation officer who would talk about some problem that was not very acute or difficult. Nevertheless, I listened carefully and tried to be helpful. After a while, I began to get a feeling that the officers were overburdened and that some of them feared that ventilating their concerns about their most difficult cases would cause the dam of problems to break open, leaving them overwhelmed and unable to carry on. This may have been one reason why each of the officers who came to see me discussed cases which were not difficult or pressing. Gradually I sensed that perhaps the problems they presented were similar to, but milder than, the problems in those cases that were extremely disturbing to them.

The officers in the boys' division reported their difficulties with hostile and violent delinquents. They gradually began to describe their fear of these youngsters, fear which they felt they had to hide. They believed it necessary to behave with these youngsters as if the fear did not exist. They also began to describe some of their retaliatory and punitive feelings.

For the most part, the young officers, who were recently out of college and bore their psychology courses freshly in mind, tried to win over the adolescents by their sympathetic, good-Joe, and big-brother attitudes, hoping by these methods to reduce and avoid the boys' hostility and aggressiveness. They overlooked and excused missed appointments. They ignored, or were ignorant of, the lies, deceptions, and half truths communicated by the probationers and their parents. Often they sensed the truth but felt uneasy about facing the parents and the youth with this knowledge. Some seemed blind to the evidence of petty thievery, truancy, and other delinquency. In a few instances, they ignored all of the signs of impending major delinquencies as the youngsters became more insolent in their attitudes toward the officer and more indifferent about keeping appointments. They failed to make inquiries which would have revealed flagrant violation of the terms of probation, especially those requiring regular attendance at school, obedience to the curfew, and no socializing with former gang members. Then, after the major delinquency or crime was committed, they would express righteous anger for being deceived after having trusted the youth. Frequently, an officer in that situation would then recommend a harsh punishment unconsciously designed to get the youngster out of his hair.

In consultation, it became clear that some officers resented the fact that the probationers were not punished by the courts for their misdeeds. Several said that their fathers would have beaten them for such behavior, and they recommended beating as the only way to cure the delinquent. Nevertheless, when relating the particular delinquencies and crimes of their probationers, the same persons often made comments like, "Man, it took guts to do that," or "Boy, what a sharp operator that guy is!" In these instances, one could sense the vicarious identification with the delinquent which made work with him difficult. The officers' contacts with their probationers' parents, some of whom were indifferent, apathetic, or delinquent themselves, occasioned comments like, "It's that kid's old man and old lady that need the beating," or, "This kid's folks don't even know he's alive." A few stated that the attitude of their probationers' parents sometimes reminded them of experiences with their own parents.

As the consultation became helpful to a few officers, more of them wanted to present their cases to me. Later, the supervisors began to attend, and finally they began to plan the conferences so they could be present when their staff discussed cases.

THE PROBATION OFFICER'S FEAR OF FEELINGS

In consultation, as I began to pick up the unspoken fear that a few officers had of their probationers, I described the kinds of feelings I knew these adolescents produced in people. Sometimes I related an experience of mine where I had been forced to recognize and admit my own fear. For example, one day when I was in the military service, a psychotic paratrooper stormed into my office on the ward and demanded the morphine he'd had at other hospitals. My corpsmen stood around terrified, and I could not hide my own fear in the face of this huge, menacing soldier. I knew he'd been riding roughshod over the nurses and corpsmen, all of whom were afraid of him. Despite my fear I knew I had to take a stand. I told him that I was scared as hell of him and that I knew he could tear me apart, but that no matter what he did, as a physician I could not give him a drug I felt was dangerous to him when I knew he needed other medication. He glared at me malevolently for what seemed many minutes, and I tried to keep my shaking head steady to meet his gaze. Slowly he lowered his eyes and asked, "Well, what do you think would help me?" I prescribed a sedative, which he took, and that was the turning point on the ward. Subsequently, he became fairly cooperative, took medication, and seemed more relaxed.

My purpose in telling this and other anecdotes was to help the officers feel that, by admitting and expressing their fears of their probationers, they might be less burdened by them and eventually might find a way of dealing with them through close attention to the tasks confronting the officer when dealing with such delinquent youth.

The unconscious factors which led to such fears and desires to appease their probationers were not discussed. Instead, we began to talk about what kinds of experiences these youngsters must have had to bring them to delinquency. I especially pointed out how parents who were unconcerned or who behaved erratically sometimes ignored, or even encouraged, their child's predelinquent acts if these acts could relieve them of the responsibility of giving personal attention to the child. I used the experiences recounted by the officers to show how the tendency to ignore signs or hunches about violation of probation, along with lack of vigilance and firmness in playing these hunches, could make it appear that they did not value the delinquent (just as fear and indifference had produced the same effect in the parent-child relationship) and could encourage repetition or continuation of the child's delinquent behavior pattern.

Some children use delinquent behavior as a means of compelling adults to behave in an authoritative and concerned way toward them. In my own experience, an adult who fails to understand or recognize signs of impending destructive or antisocial behavior is himself delinquent. The adult's failure to act promptly and firmly once he is aware of such signs—because he vainly hopes that nothing more will occur—usually results in the execution of the dreaded acts. One time in my own home, for example, I made the mistake of not putting down a book in which I was absorbed, getting up from my chair, and putting a stop immediately to some potentially destructive behavior by my youngsters. A few minutes later they broke a lamp. When I reacted with vehement anger, one of them remarked: "You knew this would happen, didn't you? Why didn't you stop us before it was too late?" He was correct. Although I sensed that inevitably something would be broken, I still hoped that nothing would happen. Most officers were able to relate similar experiences from their own work.

I gave many other examples of being "conned" or taken in, and of trusting a youngster's insincere promises against my better judgment, with the inevitable recurrence of trouble. To illustrate how vigilance and prompt action may help a delinquent, I told of my early experience as a child psychiatrist with a delinquent eleven-year-old who was in the hospital. This youngster, was so sly and clever that he could maneuver other children into stealing or violence without putting himself in a position to be caught. Whenever he was accused, his wide-eyed innocence would enrage the staff. One day we decided with the nursing staff that we'd hold him responsible for every antisocial act on the ward; no matter who the culprit was, we'd isolate this eleven-year-old or take away his privileges. We frankly admitted that this policy might be unfair to him; but because we were convinced this would be helpful to him, we were prepared to take the risks. After a few days of using this technique for every disturbance on the ward, this smooth-talking, hard, self-assured youngster became jumpy and anxious; he pleaded with others to maintain order and for the first time participated eagerly in all the ward chores instead of bossing the other youngsters. As his usual methods of dealing with people and of evading the consequences of his actions no longer served him, he also became more amenable to psychotherapy and began to improve.

When delinquent youngsters and their parents meet (perhaps for the first time) an adult whose firmness in dealing with irregularities and falsehoods is consistent and continuous, they are usually compelled to behave somewhat differently.

Thus, the officers and I discussed how the dynamic principles of authoritative, but nonauthoritarian and nonretaliatory behavior will alter delinquent character structure. These discussions seemed to help them see their tasks in a somewhat different and clearer light, and do their jobs more effectively with less stress.

Understanding Sexual Misbehavior

Women officers whose charges were usually sexually promiscuous as well as antisocial also were helped. A few of them were, overtly, coldly disapproving of the girls' sexual behavior; unconsciously, they envied them. The envy was evidenced by angry, hostile comments about the girls' sexual freedom and their lack of responsibility for the children resulting from their promiscuous relationships. Eventually it became clear that the officers' covert hostility was alienating the girls, who had used sex as a means of feeling emotionally close to, and wanted by, someone. Thus, the officers were unable to establish the type of relationship that could sustain the girls in school and jobs. In several instances, officers who were overtly solicitous with these girls were still not particularly helpful to them. It became evident in the course of discussion of these cases that the solicitude—i.e., the "you poor dear" attitude— was also hostile and deprecating, and indicated that the officer felt superior to the girl. The solicitude also seemed to be another way of denying the fact that such sexual impulses and behavior were human and part of the officer's emotional experience. The probationers spotted the phoniness and gave these particular officers an especially bad time.

The officers found it helpful to discuss possible reasons for the girls' sexual acting-out and for their brittle "I couldn't care less" attitudes. Using various illustrations, we repeatedly discussed how difficult it was to feel friendly, interested, and helpful in the face of these girls' challenges, defiance, and indifference. While we never talked about the officers' unconscious envy of the girls' acting-out of sexual impulses, we did talk about the experiences of persons in other fields who have to deal with disturbing sexual behavior. Our culture, our upbringing, and our resulting sexual attitudes make it difficult for us to feel easy about impulsive and overt sexual behavior. The fact that sexual activity is often used to express other feelings, desires, and needs is therefore difficult for us to understand. When underlying feelings are misunderstood, the offensive behavior is not dealt with clearly. After a while, several of the officers began to talk about their probationers with more understanding, and their relationships with the girls changed markedly. One of the supervisors seemed to find these discussions especially useful and was subsequently able to help her own workers with many of their problems.

Attitudes Toward Parents

Some of the officers in the protective and adoptive services division were especially handicapped by their anger toward, and resentment of, the neglectful, indifferent, helpless parents, who— as it became clear from their comments—represented parental figures out of their own past. After consultation, several were able to find strengths in some of the parents. They were also able to understand the difficulties and dilemmas of foster and adoptive parents of difficult youngsters. When we began to explore what made parents behave as they did, how deprivations during the parents' own childhood affected their capacities, this group of officers seemed to feel less anger toward the parents with whom they worked. I described the experience that other child psychiatrists and I have had of overidentifying with the child until we were able to learn, from direct work with the troubled parents, that they were not the monsters we judged them to be from our work with the child alone. As we gathered data on some of the serious deprivations suffered by the parents—deprivations which made it difficult and sometimes impossible for them to give very much to a child—the officers seemed to understand the parents' problems more clearly.

RESULTS OF CONSULTATION

Consultation once or twice a month for several years helped a number of probation officers with some of the most difficult problems imposed by their job. Their increased firmness, vigilance, and promptness of action seemed to make the total job easier. Several workers reported that, through the insights gained in consultation, they were able to use the probationers' reactions to their attentive vigilance as a means of assessing and then selecting those who might benefit most from more intensive work. Increased efforts with these youngsters began to pay off.

Supervisors who participated in consultation sessions became aware of those attitudes and methods used by the consultant which seemed most helpful to the staff. They began to apply these methods, with gratifying results.

As a consequence of the workers' and supervisors' experiences, the chief probation officer began to realize the possible value of consultation and started telling me of various administrative concerns, his problems with several supervisors in the agency, and his relations with the juvenile court judge. He then went on to review carefully the job of the supervisors and subsequently decided that requiring them to carry a heavy caseload of probationers in addition to supervising staff was unrealistic. The judge, who had made increasingly favorable comments about the work of the department, began to listen more carefully to the chief probation officer's requests for additional staff to do a better and more thorough job, and gave more active support to the requested budgetary increases. Subsequently, the board of supervisors granted an increase which made possible the hiring of more probation officers.

In analyzing with the chief probation officer the part that consultation played in bringing about this long desired and frequently requested budgetary increase, we clarified several important developments:

First, as the probation officers were helped to work more thoroughly and efficiently, they could begin to assess how much of their time was required to do an effective job. They and their supervisors could then estimate the caseload size which permitted such thorough work—not in terms of ideals set up by the probation authorities but in terms of actual experience. Once the probation officers could keep up with their load, they could present the true dimensions of the problem to the judge and the county board of supervisors.

Second, just as teachers are burdened with certain unrealistic expectations—that they must love all children, that as surrogate parents they must make up for the lack of love or character attributes not provided by the actual parents—so are workers in juvenile probation departments. In our culture, parents and their substitutes decry, abhor, and deal harshly with violence, antisocial behavior, defiance of authority, sexual misbehavior, etc. Yet, we are educated by magazines, movies, and television, to admire, envy, and applaud such acts. The father who preaches obedience to law and respect for authority may be sadistically cruel in punishing his child. The mother who teaches virtue, chastity, and purity may avidly and continually be gossiping about the sexual behavior of her neighbors. This division of feeling, both conscious and unconscious, complicates the job of the probation officer. It may lead him to be excessively harsh in order to defend himself against such envy of, or identification with, the probationer's behavior, or to be excessively placating and ineffectual because of the fears and anxiety presented by these ambivalent feelings.

It is in reducing the general strains and burdens imposed by these conflicts that the mental health consultant in a probation department finds his reward and satisfaction.

LEARNING MENTAL HEALTH CONSULTATION:
HISTORY AND PROBLEMS*

I. N. Berlin

Mental health consultation as a means of helping professional workers in caretaking agencies to function more effectively is a relatively recent development. Papers on consultation to agencies first appeared in the literature of the 1930's and with increasing frequency, in the 1940's. The consultant's role in agencies was seen as one of providing technical advice or of educating the workers, as Goldman's (13) 1940 paper illustrates. Sloane (21), in 1936, described a method in which the consultant helped untrained social workers to deal with difficult clients by the consultants' retention of case responsibility and concerted efforts to educate the worker to a higher level of functioning.

The first paper to deal with mental health consultation as it is now conceived was written by Jules Coleman (12) in 1947. Coleman's paper on psychiatric consultation in casework agencies stressed the following: (1) The consultant's chief concern is not the worker's case or client but an understanding of why the worker presents this problem now. (2) His object is to discover how the worker needs help and which of the worker's feelings need to be understood and dealt with. (3) The consultant, unlike the supervisor, does not represent the agency and is therefore concerned with the worker and his problems, not with how the case is handled.

In 1950 Susselman (22), in a paper on psychiatric consultation in a probation department, described how the consultant's awareness that the consultee's work problems were often internalized conflicts could be used to help the consultee by clearly presenting and discussing with him the dynamically appropriate alternatives for these critical problems. (See page 167 of this volume.)

---

*Reprinted with permission from Mental Hygiene, 48:257-266, 1964.

That same year Maddux (16), using Coleman's methods, described how relatively untrained public welfare workers could be helped to function more effectively if the consultant understood what caused their anxiety. Problems indigenous to a particular agency, such as handling the dependency of clients in public welfare agencies, or specific difficulties in dealing with people which the worker might have because of lack of training, knowledge, or personal problems—all need to be understood as possible contributors to anxiety. Maddux saw the consultant's job to be that of relieving the worker's anxiety by means of ventilation of his feelings of anger, hostility, rejection, etc., to a noncritical, nonjudgmental consultant who does not become involved in personal problems but looks at these difficulties as professional problems. He also indicated that he found little need to give direct suggestion or advice, which tended to make the worker dependent. Some six years later I described similar findings based on my experiences in a variety of agencies (2).

The concept of mental health consultation that comes close to the one most workers find helpful has been enunciated best by Caplan (8,10,11,19). Although Caplan includes a variety of activities under his category of mental health consultation, his emphasis is on the consultant's understanding of the consultee's troubles as being the result of the worker's intrapsychic conflicts, upon which the client's problems and behavior impinge. The technique of helping the consultee is an indirect one; it uses the difficulties and problems of the client as a focus for discussion. This delimits the problem as a work problem, relieves anxiety, and helps the consultee resolve similar problems of his own.

Out of many different settings and experiences in the last ten or twelve years, a number of other workers have contributed to the refinement and expansion of the specialized techniques known as mental health consultation (1,3,4,6,7,17,20).

TRAINING IN CONSULTATION

Several formal centers for training in consultation have developed. The pioneering effort at Harvard by Gerald Caplan has been a great stimulus to mental health consultation throughout the country, since the training program has also provided opportunities to test hypotheses and to further research work. Viola Bernard at Columbia University's School of Public Health has developed a curriculum geared to training psychiatrists in community psychiatry, one phase of which is supervised training in consultation.

In the last several years Portia Hume has directed a new Center for Training in Community Psychiatry, under the auspices of the California Department of Mental Hygiene, in Berkeley. Here also there is heavy emphasis on seminars and supervised training in mental health consultation. Several training programs in general psychiatry and child psychiatry include some orientation and training in mental health consultation. Many agencies are also conducting in-service training programs in consultation (9,14,23).

My efforts over the last twelve years to teach mental health consultation to social workers and psychologists in two school systems, and to child psychiatrists in training, have made me aware of some repetitive obstacles to the learning of mental health consultation that require special attention by the teacher. I was particularly encouraged to find that a colleague and pioneer in mental health consultation and its teaching, Beulah Parker, had recently written about the need for supervision to meet some of these problems (18).

The Mental Health Consultation Process

Mental health consultation can be described as a process in which a consultant tries to help a consultee from another profession with a work problem. Learning this process may be difficult, especially for those mental health professionals already experienced in their generic practices.

The method involves a diagnostic appraisal of the conflicts which cause the consultee's work problem; dynamic understanding of the anxieties and of the form in which they are presented to the consultant; assessment of the integrative capacities of the consultee; efforts to reduce his anxieties by appropriate comments which indicate the consultant's understanding of, acceptance of, and personal experience with, similar feelings; illumination of conflicts engendered in the consultee by the behavior of his clients; and, finally, discussion of how similar problems have been handled by others so that the consultee can see how he might deal with the problem he presents.

The consultee often identifies with the consultant's attitudes toward the consultee's troubles and anxieties, and sometimes with the methods by which the consultant deals with them. Thus, the consultant needs to have clearly in mind that his attitudes and behavior often provide a model for the consultee (5).

The mental health professional—social worker, psychologist, or psychiatrist—who begins to learn consultation methods must unlearn some of his traditional ways of working with people (18). In this process the consultee is a collaborator, not a patient, client, or counselee. His personal psychopathology is not the focus of discussion, which means that the mental health professional requires considerable reorientation. Since the process is an indirect one, it is often slow. The results may not be evident for a long time, and then perhaps are recognized only in the reduced need for consultation. Thus, the satisfactions and rewards of individual psychotherapeutic efforts are often not present.

Even more than in individual work, when the process is effective, the consultee may matter-of-factly accept the improvement in his work, sometimes not being aware of how he has been helped. When he is aware, he may not acknowledge it to the consultant. Since the usual ways of gauging one's effectiveness and usefulness are missing, at critical moments it is often difficult for the consultant to refrain from using the tried and true methods of individual psychotherapy. The result is usually an increase of problems in consultation.

My own experience has shown that those workers who have had training and practice in psychotherapeutic work with children and parents learn consultation practice more readily. They have long ago learned to hear—in the complaints of the parent about the other parent or the child—disguised statements about the immediate patient. Therefore, in consultation they can hear in the consultee's statements about his concern with a client what he is saying about himself.

Problems in Initiating Consultation

The contract in any consultation which is to be an ongoing process may present problems because it may be honored in different ways. In all varieties of individual psychotherapy, the understanding at the beginning of the work forms the framework for treatment. At least the person seeking help agrees to certain appointment times and fees, and commits himself to try to talk about his troubles.

In consultation where there is no crisis, the initial agreement may be ignored; the time, place, and conditions of consultation may seem never to have been talked about. The consultant is then faced with defining the conditions of consultation by his own attitudes and behavior with the consultee. His efforts to help the consultee with the obstacles to his keeping the contract may be a necessary demonstration of the consultation process, and vital to the development of the consultation relationship. The consultant may find himself initially giving lectures to staff or doing much direct service as part of developing the relationship.

In one instance a principal asked the consultant to do a different kind of task each time—i.e., interview a child or a parent, visit a classroom, make a referral, give a speech to the PTA, etc.—until he finally became convinced that the consultant really was concerned with understanding and helping the administrator, and was

not another prima donna from the superintendent's office concerned only with his special little project and his own professionally
narcissistic satisfactions.

Normal Anxiety in Consultation

Each mental health profession has its traditional roles and attitudes for reducing the practitioner's anxieties in dealing with the
patient. The role of the person asking for help is also fairly clearly delineated. Thus, the self-expectations and expectations of the
other person are quite clear. In consultation, however, there is no
traditional role and no clear expectation of consultee and consultant. In fact, in any consultation session one may be faced with
unpredictable crises and demands for their solution; unsolvable
problems may be presented in which the etiological factors are
unknowable for the time being, and understanding of the consultee's
troubles and their meaning at that moment may be impossible to
achieve.

As one colleague so clearly put it, anxiety is to be taken for
granted as a part of the consultant's expected experience in most
consultation sessions (15). The fact that opportunities to understand and to become familiar with a particular consultee's methods of handling problems requires a fairly long experience together
may burden the consultant with a great deal of uncertainty and
anxiety for a long period of time. On the other hand, when one
learns to accept the uncertainty as part of the process, the
attendant anxiety is reduced. In its place comes a feeling of anticipation and pleasure in the creative application of one's knowledge,
perception, and intuition. It does make consultation stimulating,
and may evoke from the consultant and consultee creative solutions
to problems and constant growth in self-understanding and understanding of the consultative process.

The Introductory Phase of Consultation

The honeymoon is a phase of the get-acquainted period which
occurs in most relationships and which is a recognized and
reckoned-with part of psychotherapeutic work. Most therapists
look at this period as an interval between the patient's effort to
establish a good impression on first meeting a new person, and the
time when his resistances and characteristic modes of dealing with
meaningful people in his life assert themselves.

In the consultation process the honeymoon period is especially
trying and deceptive; overtly everything may seem to be going well,
but covertly the consultee is complaining to superiors and colleagues that consultation is a waste of time and a lot of humbug.

Often the more anxious and insecure the consultee, the greater the discrepancy between the overt and covert communications.

Thus, the trainee-consultant may be completely surprised and devastated when he hears the complaints. He may find it difficult, then, to deal with the consultee about the complaints in such a way as to clarify and strengthen the consultation relationship. At such a point it is usually not easy to assess anew the past work in consultation, to understand where and why one has missed cues, and what one has not understood of the consultee's problems.

Furthermore, effective consultation may evoke anxiety and complaining which reflects the particular reality situation about which neither the consultant nor anyone else can effect change. Only continued consultation might reduce the consultee's turmoil. As in the matter of the original contract, the consultant's efforts to explore dissatisfactions, his ability to be nondefensive and to admit mistakes, his honest and earnest desire to be of help, may solidify the consultation relationship as a result of such "honeymoon" problems; this might otherwise take many, many more months of consultation to achieve.

The Theme in Consultation Sessions*

Colleagues and students who have been present in consultation sessions with various agencies have often remarked that they would be more active than I in consultation, i.e., reply to more questions or respond to more implicit requests and demands. They have additionally commented that they noticed that after I listened for some time, my comments often did not seem to answer directly the consultees' queries and demands, and yet seemed to help them, often relieved anxiety, and resulted in the consultees' functioning more effectively on their job, as was borne out by subsequent meetings.

I have come in the past ten years to recognize that the consultee or group of consultees usually present work problems which reflect neurotic conflicts. These conflicts, in my experience, express themselves in a central theme during the consultation session. I have therefore learned to wait until I could form a hypothesis about the nature of the conflict theme and until such a hypothesis was validated by the continued comments of the consultee. I have found that only then could I respond relevantly and helpfully to the consultee. This is not to say that comments and interaction by the consultant may not help the consultee state the theme more clear-

---

*This section is reprinted with permission from the American Journal of Orthopsychiatry, 30:827-828, 1960.

192

ly. Thus in a recent school consultation about a defiant, provocative, hostile adolescent boy, the questions and demands that
administrators and teachers put to the "expert" centered around
how this boy should be handled. As it evolved, the theme of the
group was their conflicts about the amount of anger, hate, and
retaliatory feeling he aroused in all of them, which prevented their
working with him effectively. Thus it was only when those feelings
were dealt with, and exclusion from school was mentioned by the
consultant as one possible outcome of the conference, that they
were able to discuss methods by which the youngster could be
helped.

Consultation with Administrators

While most of the foregoing comments apply to ongoing or
continuous consultation in general—as contrasted with crisis
consultation—they have a particular bearing on mental health
consultation with agency administrators. In my experience this
is the most difficult and trying aspect of consultation to learn and,
therefore, to teach.

The administrator's position makes him especially sensitive
and vulnerable to a threat arising from his handling of problems
that involve authority, status, or his possible failure to deal with
any difficulties concerning clients or staff. As a result, many
administrators feel they must never appear—especially to their
superiors — to be in need of help in solving problems. Often they
also feel that they must not admit to any mental health professional
that he might have knowledge or techniques which could be useful
in dealing with their problems.

One consultant found that while a school administrator made
relevant referrals and seemed to appreciate help in understanding
and working with parents, she also felt any regular meetings would
be an acknowledgment that she was not a self-sufficient, completely
competent administrator. It was only when this administrator's
help was enlisted as a collaborator (in preventive mental health
evaluations of children and in helping her teachers to be more
effective in understanding, evaluating, and using educative methods
to help some of these very young, potentially disturbed children)
that she could accept regular work with the consultant and eventually discuss a few of her problems as an administrator.

One of the most difficult problems in consultation, especially
with school administrators—although this is true also of some
other agency heads—stems from the combination of realistic pressures, which keep them constantly busy and unavailable, and their
relative autonomy in the school. This makes it possible for a few
administrators to shift their responsibilities to subordinates; thus

they provide little actual leadership in the school, and yet they prevent the subordinates from operating effectively with other administrative personnel by fragmenting their authority.

In one instance the responsibilities were divided between vice-principal and head counselor so that neither had complete authority to handle a disturbed child; and whenever they made any effort to get together to map out methods of working together, the administrator would redefine the responsibilities for each person and defeat every effort to solve a difficult problem. In the resulting chaos, the principal would severely criticize each subordinate for falling down on the job, take matters into his own hands, and exclude the youngster from school.

In another instance, an administrator had seemed to promote jealousy among his very bright and competent subordinates, and kept them divided so that they were unable to work together as a team to solve pressing agency problems. Apparent anxiety about his job made these divisive efforts necessary so that he would feel less threatened. He repeatedly stated that despite his best efforts he could not get his subordinates to work together in solving the agency's problems.

The pressures incumbent in the job make it possible for the anxious administrator to be always too busy to sit down with the consultant for very long. Clients, staff, visitors, and various meetings come first. These pressures also permit ostensibly legitimate demands to be made in terms of urgent referrals, direct service, etc., and may make it impossible for the consultant and administrator to meet to discuss other problems.

One of the most frequent problems consultants encounter with public agency administrators stems from their conviction that they must undertake every assignment given to them, carry out every suggestion made by superiors, and never say "no" to any demands from the community. These administrators are literally over-whelmed, and often frightened at the enormity of their job and the fact that they can see no relief in sight.

Another difficult problem for the student learning consultation techniques is the administrator who responds to the consultant's attitude of expertness by handing all his problems over to him for solution. He often demands constant reassurance from the consultant as well. Such administrators, and they are relatively few, react to the consultant's confidence and aura of competence, and especially to his ready and helpful suggestions, with regressive helplessness, as if they could not possibly exist unless the consultant remained constantly at their side to advise and help them.

Another very difficult aspect of learning consultation with administrators comes from the fact that sometimes one's most effective consultative work is most threatening to them. This is especially so in the kind of continuous consultation I teach, where the administrator is present at consultation with his subordinates (5). He can thus sanction any action that comes from consultation, but most important, as he is exposed to the consultation process, he can slowly learn by identification with the consultant how he may more effectively help his own subordinates with their problems.

If the consultant is not clearly aware of the administrator's anxities and competitive feelings with the consultant, he may attend only to the worker's problems and, through his a curate and precise understanding of the subordinate's problems, help him with such apparent ease that the administrator may feel impotent and worthless because he had failed to help his worker. Thus the consultative relationship may be jeopardized. It s therefore necessary, although difficult, for the mental heal consultant to learn to think on many levels at once, not only ab ut the dynamics of the individual in front of him, but also about the dynamics of the entire agency and its varied personnel. This is no small task.

We have delineated at length some of the difficulties in mental health consultation with administrators so that consultants may become aware of how long it may take to overcome some of these obstacles and may realize that in each situation one needs to give oneself sufficient time to get to know the people involved; then one can begin to understand the particular anxieties and conflicts manifested in each of these difficult situations.

From such an assessment one can plan how and where the consultant's behavior, attitudes, and help to specific persons in the agency hierarchy might begin to reduce some of the tensions and shift the forces in the direction of more integrative functioning of the staff.

Since the consultant's purpose is to help the administrator to do his own job more effectively, the consultant must learn not to respond to helplessness by taking over administrative functions or decisions, since these are not his job. Nor should he participate in intra-agency strife by siding with either the divisive administrator or his impotent-feeling subordinates. Here the consultant begins to learn that divisiveness on the part of the administrator signals his need for help and support in certain areas of his professional work.

Consultation Versus Direct Service

I should also mention that in trying to help mental health consultants learn consultation I have become aware of the struggle each consultant has about whether consultation is as effective a way of helping an agency as direct service. Of course, one of the

vital factors is that the satisfactions inherent in doing direct service are not often forthcoming in consultation for a long time.
Direct service, where the consultant does for the consultee what
he needs to learn to do for himself, is also usually more promptly
relieving and satisfying to the consultee. Thus, learning consultation may require, in addition to the vicissitudes of mastering a
new skill, a delay both in personal gratification from the work and
in satisfying the demands of the agency.

Levels of Communication in Requests for Help

The previously mentioned need to be attuned to many levels of
communication is difficult to learn and to use effectively. Thus,
each request for help may carry both a plea for aid and a warning
that to act on the request is tantamount to saying to the administrator that he is not adequate. When, for example, a principal
asks the consultant to go to work with a teacher about a problem
child, unless the worker understands this request as a possible
question about whose job it really is to help the teacher, the action
of the consultant may disrupt the consultation relationship.

The consultant tries to make clear to the administrator by his
attitudes that his job as an expert is to help the administrator with
the mental health aspects of his job. In recent years difficult
mental health problems are more often being presented to agency
workers and thus to administrators. The need for help from
mental health experts is correspondingly greater.

Requests from administrators for help or understanding of
troubles are sometimes very indirect and vague. These requests
need to be understood and handled by the consultant as an opportunity for some mutual appraisal of the request with the administrator. It is usually most helpful to react to an indirect request
as an appeal for help to a subordinate about his problems with a
client, rather than appeal for help by the administrator for his
own problems.

Despite the many difficulties in learning to consult with administrators, I've come to feel that the time thus invested is far more
productive in helping staff and clients than any other kind of mental
health service.

SOME PROBLEMS IN THE TEACHING OF CONSULTATION

Anticipation of some of the most frequent anxieties and frustrations, hopefully, may reduce the feeling of failure in the trainee.
Consultation vignettes presented to illustrate the common problems seem to be quite effective. Students have told of how they

have recalled such vignettes at times of extreme frustration and
have been able to view the situation a bit more objectively.

Process recordings of consultation sessions are valuable for
the delineation of dynamics of consultation. Such recording makes
possible an understanding of the subtleties of the consultation
interaction that is not possible when the trainee relies on his
memory. Supervisory meetings held with a skilled supervisor at
least once a week are most helpful—probably essential—to learning consultation.

I have found it difficult to help some trainees not to use con-
frontation techniques when these skilled and previously effective
mental health professionals find themselves hamstrung by consultees who avoid them, forget the meetings, or complain to
colleagues about the failure of the consultant to be very helpful.
On rare occasions it has been necessary for the trainee to use his
therapeutic skills on the consultee so that he may experience first-
hand the reaction of the consultee who feels he is being treated as
a patient. Usually some role-playing by the supervisor, when he
understands the meaning of the consultee's behavior in a particular
instance, permits the trainee to observe how the consultee might
react to various approaches.

The student-consultant's failure to engage the administrator-
consultee in meaningful consultative work, because of the time it
often takes to bring about engagement, may leave the student feeling inept and futile. Such experiences may make the trainee certain that this process is inefficient or ineffectual. I have found
that it is easier to help the trainee persist in his efforts if there
are several trainees, at the same point in their training, who can
share their mutual frustrations and recognize that this is a regular, predictable phase in the consultation process.

The rewards in teaching consultation come when the trainee
has been able to work through the many difficulties, and can
finally see the results of his efforts in the more effective work
of the administrator with his staff, and of the staff with their
clients. I have come to feel that the trainee has mastered consultation practice when he begins to find fun and anticipatory excitement in consultation meetings; and when he follows his
intuitive leads to realize the creative possibilities in mental
health consultation.

REFERENCES

1. BABCOCK, C. Some observations in consultative experience. Soc. Serv. Rev., 23:347-57, 1949.

2. BERLIN, I. N. Some learning experiences as psychiatric consultant in the schools. Ment. Hygiene, 40:215-36, 1956. Reprinted in I. N. Berlin & S. A. Szurek (Eds.), Learning and its disorders. Vol. 1, the Langley Porter Child Psychiatry Series. Palo Alto, Calif.: Science and Behavior Books, 1965.

3. BERLIN, I. N. The theme in mental health consultation sessions. Amer. J. Orthopsychiat., 30:827-828, 1960. (See page 191 of this volume.)

4. BERLIN, I. N. Mental health consultation in schools as a means of communicating mental health principles. J. Amer. Acad. Child Psychiat., 1:671-79, 1962. (See page 199 of this volume.)

5. BERLIN, I. N. Psychiatric consultation on the antidelinquency project. Calif. J. second. Educ., 35:198-202, 1960. Reprinted in I. N. Berlin & S. A. Szurek (Eds.), Learning and its disorders. Vol. 1, the Langley Porter Child Psychiatry Series. Palo Alto, Calif.: Science and Behavior Books, 1965.

6. BETTELHEIM, B., et al. Psychiatric consultation in residential treatment. Amer. J. Orthopsychiat., 28:256-90, 1958.

7. BINDMAN, A. J. Mental health consultation theory and practice. J. consult. Psychol., 23:473-82, 1959.

8. CAPLAN, G. Concepts of mental health and consultation. Washington, D.C.: U. S. Children's Bureau, 1959.

9. CAPLAN, G. An approach to the education of community mental health specialists. Ment. Hygiene, 43:268-80, 1962.

10. CAPLAN, G. Mental health consultation in schools. In The elements of a community mental health program. New York: Milbank Memorial Fund, 1956.

11. CAPLAN, G. Principles of mental health consultation. Unpublished manuscript.

12. COLEMAN, J. R. Psychiatric consultation in casework agencies. Amer. J. Orthopsychiat., 17:533-39, 1947.

13. GOLDMAN, G. The psychiatrist and the function of the private agency. Amer. J. Orthopsychiat., 10:548-66, 1940.

14. KAZANJIAN, V., STEIN, S., & WEINBERG, W. L. An introduction to mental health consultation. Public Health Monograph #69. Washington, D.C.: U. S. Public Health Service, 1962.

15. LAMBERT, N. Personal communication.

16. MADDUX, J. F. Psychiatric consultation in a public welfare agency. Amer. J. Orthopsychiat., 20:754-64, 1950.

17. PARKER, B. Psychiatric consultation to non-psychiatric professional workers. Public Health Monograph #53. Washington, D.C.: U. S. Public Health Service, 1958.

18. PARKER, B. The value of supervision in training psychiatrists for mental health consultation. Ment. Hygiene, 45:94-100, 1961.

19. ROSENFELD, J. M., & CAPLAN, G. Techniques of staff consultation in an immigrant children's organization in Israel. Amer. J. Orthopsychiat.

20. SIEGEL, D. Consultation: Some guiding principles. New York: Family Service Association of America, 1955.

21. SLOANE, P. The use of a consultation method in casework therapy. Amer. J. Orthopsychiat., 6:355-61, 1936.

22. SUSSELMAN, S. The role of the psychiatrist in a probation agency. Focus, 29:33, 1950. (See page 167 of this volume.)

23. VON FELSINGER, J. M., & KLEIN, D. C. Professional training for the mental health field. Ment. Hygiene, 46:203-17, 1962.

MENTAL HEALTH CONSULTATION IN SCHOOLS
AS A MEANS OF COMMUNICATING
MENTAL HEALTH PRINCIPLES*

I. N. Berlin

The mental health consultant in a school system has a unique opportunity to communicate and sometimes to demonstrate mental health principles to teachers. Perhaps the most important principle he can communicate is the fact that all human feelings can be talked about without shame, blame, or passing judgment on the teacher as a bad person. By his attitude of concern, attentiveness, and respect, the consultant demonstrates his relationship to the teacher as a professional colleague, and so indicates that the teacher's problems, with their attendant mixed feelings, are of mutual concern. The consultant's encouragement of verbal expression by the teacher of all his feelings about his work is greatly enhanced, in my experience, as the consultant progressively clarifies that he is not there to analyze the teacher, to pry into hidden motivations, or to uncover skeletons in the teacher's personal closet. He demonstrates in many ways that his job as an expert in interpersonal relations is to help the teacher understand himself in terms of the job he is doing, and, in particular, to help him to be consciously aware of his feelings about the particular child who is a problem for him. The purpose is always to enable the teacher to do his work more effectively.

Another mental health principle the consultant can demonstrate effectively is that every person has limitations, both professionally and personally. Unreal self-expectations and their aftermaths of tension and exhaustion from increasing conflict may seriously inter-

---

*Reprinted with permission from The Journal of the American Academy of Child Psychiatry, 1:671–679, 1962.

fere with teaching. Thus the understanding, acceptance, and assessment of one's own limitations are important for good mental health.

A third vital principle that can be demonstrated by the consultant centers around authority. Workers in a hierarchical setting need to be able to accept constituted authority and to work under regulations without undue conflict. This may be especially important for mental health when, as sometimes occurs, the authority is unjust and the regulations are restrictive. Rebellion and its attendant repercussions in the teacher's teaching frequently only increase the tensions between teachers and administrators.

Two experiences illustrate the consultant's role in demonstrating the mental health principle that all feelings aroused by a pupil can be talked about. A third-grade teacher and her principal asked to talk with me about a non-learning Negro youngster whose size and aggressiveness made him a terror, both in the classroom and out of it. The principal described the boy's behavior in the classroom and school yard, and the difficulties the teacher and the administrator encountered in handling the boy. While the principal talked, the teacher sat by very quietly and appeared frozen. When asked to add her comments to the principal's, she remarked in a barely audible voice that it had all been said, and sat stiffly in her chair. As I began to comment about what a handful this must be for the teacher to contend with all day, and that we psychiatrists were pretty lucky because at the worst we had to deal with such a child for only an hour once or twice a week, the teacher grinned tightly.

I then talked about a learning experience of my own, of which this child had reminded me. This was a severely hostile, aggressive ten-year-old boy who presented a constant dilemma in the early weeks of treatment. If I tried to stop him from attacking me and breaking up the playroom before he got started, he accused me of jumping him before he had done anything; and I felt guilty and uncomfortable about being unfair to such a disturbed child. If I waited until things did get started, it required all my efforts to contain him; and I became full of mounting rage and revengeful feelings as I struggled to prevent him from hurting me or destroying equipment. In one treatment hour, after seven or eight sessions, I found myself full of murderous fury at having been hurt by him and finally having to hold this ten-year-old down on the floor with a scissor-lock around his legs and an arm-lock on his arms. I was working very hard only to restrain him and not to hurt him.

Beside myself with impotent rage, I told the boy how terribly angry I felt and how I feared that the anger he provoked in me might cause me to hurt him. If that happened, I would feel very guilty and sorry. I told him further that to avoid this possibility I had just decided to restrain him the moment he even looked as

if he were about to be violent, and that I was quite prepared to be
unfair to him at times. I was determined to continue this until he
had shown me that he could begin to control himself. After three
more hours of testing and protesting as I restrained him at every
sign of incipient trouble, he began to settle down and express his
feelings through the materials in the playroom.

As I was talking, I could see the teacher's face relax; there
were little nods as I described my own feelings in the playroom
with respect to the child. When I finished, she sighed mightily and
began to talk rapidly of her own fears, the anger, the hatred, and
the helpless feelings occasioned by this boy's behavior. She
accepted my suggestion that she try to anticipate this boy's beginning unrest and stay with him, helping him do schoolwork. Her
personal attention at such moments, rather than a half hope from
a distance that the ominous signs might not bring their inevitable
result, might slowly begin to help this child. Also she might in
time aid this boy to begin to communicate his feelings in words,
and to find a way out of his tension through beginning successes in
schoolwork. On my next trip to that school about six weeks later,
the administrator commented that a great change had taken place
in the teacher. Since the consultation, in which the administrator
had participated, the teacher seemed more able to talk with him
about her problems. The boy, although still a school and classroom problem, was gradually settling down.

On another occasion, a male high school teacher, after several
conversations about other problems, recounted his difficulties with
several huge, explosive boys who seemed to dare him to stop them.
Although no weakling himself, he found himself indecisive. He
feared a fight and riot if he interfered to stop the hostile, provocative behavior, yet he felt ineffectual and at the boys' mercy if he
did not take some action. Involved in this also was his feeling that
he could not ask the administrator's help with this recurring problem lest he be thought a poor teacher. As the teacher recounted
his experiences, the dean of boys, who sat by, became more and
more uncomfortable.

My comment that this was "a hell of a fix" to find oneself in
brought a "You're not kidding" from the teacher and a nod from
the dean. I then recalled a particularly difficult situation in the
Army with a psychotic soldier who had been a wrestler as well as
a much-decorated paratrooper. He terrorized the psychotic ward
and was reigning as king when I took over the service. During the
first ward rounds he made his stand clear as he towered over me
flexing his muscles, saying, "I am running things, see." Since my
fear was evident to all in my trembling hands and legs, there seemed no point in denying it. I told this psychotic patient that I was

scared of him and of what he might be able to do physically to me, but that I could not let him run the ward; I was prepared, personally and with all the MPs in the hospital if necessary, to run it as it must be run. The man glared at me for an interminably long minute. I did my best to meet his gaze. Finally, he shrugged his shoulders and disdainfully said, "Okay, have it your way," and returned to his bed. I had felt that being painfully honest about my fear, as well as clearly demonstrating my determination to carry out my job by whatever means were necessary, had been the effective elements of this interchange.

Both teacher and dean then began to discuss how they could work together to help these youngsters settle down in the classroom. It was clear to me from the dean's avid following of my account and from his relieved look when our discussion began that he had felt as stymied as the teacher by these boys and therefore unable to be of much help. The humorous aftermath of this consultation came when the dean, weeks later, commented that this teacher now had a reputation among the tough youngsters for great fearlessness because he could admit being scared.

UNREAL SELF-EXPECTATIONS

The following illustrates how the consultant's attitudes toward others and himself may help reduce unreal self-expectations and lead to greater acceptance of realistic limitations.

A typical interchange among teachers, overheard after a group consultation is: "Well, Berlin wasn't really much help today, but it's kind of nice to hear a psychiatrist say he doesn't know something." The honest, "I don't know," or "This is out of my line," in answer to insoluble problems on matters of curriculum and other subjects in which the consultant has no special competence, seems to help others to understand that they do not have to know, and be able to cope with, everything.

In many instances this begins to help the educator to delineate his relationship to the kind of work that he can do—namely, educating. It may also make it possible for the teacher to ask for help from administrators, or to call in parents when necessary, without feeling that such a call for help is an admission of failure. Thus some problems may get attention earlier, rather than at the point of impasse when both teacher and student are so disturbed emotionally that it becomes difficult to find ways to continue work.

Despite their best efforts, teachers will sometimes fail to help a disturbed child, and they need to be able to accept such failure. The consultant's readiness to illustrate from his own experience that on occasions he too has failed to be helpful demonstrates his understanding of their problem. It seems to me to be helpful to the teacher when in his comments the consultant shows that one can fail with a clear conscience after one has literally done everything one could do within one's own present scope of knowledge and professional development. As many of us have experienced, the readiness to give up and to admit failure often frees both people in a working relationship to try again. I have often witnessed that the consultant's understanding and acceptance of the administrator's and teacher's desire to exclude a child from school, because they are at the end of their rope with the child, resulted in the teacher's relief. Thus the contemplated action about which the teacher or administrator feels some guilt is accepted as reasonable in the light of the situation which has been discussed. Often later in the same discussion, after close examination of the problems and their possible causes, the teacher has reconsidered the exclusion and has been willing to try to work with the child again.

AUTHORITY AND REBELLION

In my experience, the consultant can often demonstrate that one can accept constituted authority and its regulations even when they are unfair, and that one can find ways of working within such a framework. In my own work I have insisted that administrators be present during consultation to decide what action is to be taken after we discuss the problems involved.

Sometimes teachers are temporarily angered when the consultant does not side with their rebellion against short-sighted regulations or strongly biased administrators. In such instances, it has been possible to help some of these teachers to focus on using their energies more effectively in doing a good job of teaching and working with their pupils. As energies are withdrawn from their usually fruitless rebellion and transferred to more effective teaching, the consultant begins to recognize how often the teacher's problems with authority served other purposes. Most frequently, in my experience, such rebelliousness actually served as a rationalization for the poor job of teaching that was being done. An interesting paradox is often seen. The hostile, angry rebelliousness of many teachers does not become channeled into rational action as citizens or teachers, through the organization appropriate for such action, until they begin to teach more effectively and consequently reduce the irrational aspects of their rebellion.

A number of teachers and administrators have commented that my own acceptance of severe limitations in consultation imposed by frightened, unfriendly administrators has been of help to them. They have watched to see whether I would adhere strictly to the rules that were laid down. It became clear to them that I could and did function under these restrictions until, as a result of my behavior, the administrator felt less threatened and relaxed the restrictions. One vice-principal who later went on to an important job in another school system said that such a demonstration helped him resolve a problem he had been struggling with for years and made his advancement possible.

DISCUSSION

Mental health consultation is a term made meaningful by Gerald Caplan of the Harvard School of Public Health and used by him to describe particular consultative processes previously written about under many headings. In this process a consultant, using specific consultative methods, attempts to help a consultee whose internalized conflicts interfere with effective performance of some aspect of his job.

The dynamics of the mental health consultation process are being studied by a number of workers. This paper is concerned with the particular way in which the consultation process lends itself to the communication of certain mental health principles to the teacher and administrator, and through them to other members of the school faculty. In addition, these experiences highlight several aspects of the dynamics of mental health consultation.

The consultant demonstrates in many ways his understanding of the consultees' problems and his assessment of these as work problems. When he relates similar experiences of his own and indicates the mental health principles involved which he, an authority in interpersonal matters, also had to learn, then feelings of turmoil, hate, anger, rebellion, and self-righteousness, which were largely covert, can become more overt. As some of the defenses against the eruption of such feelings are reduced, the teacher begins to feel that his problems can be resolved and is ready to listen to the methods others have used to deal with similar problems. Frequently, a teacher who has been helped will talk frankly and eagerly with colleagues and will emphasize the mental health principles he has learned.

In my own work I have insisted on the presence of administrators at most of the consultations. It reduces opportunities for divisive comments by teachers against administrators, should they later misquote the consultant to other faculty members. An even more important reason is that in my experience the consultant is often called in because the administrator has not been able to help his teacher with some particular problems, and this may indicate some difficulties on the administrator's part in doing his job effectively. As the administrator listens to the consultative sessions, he becomes aware of the consultant's attitudes which seem to help

the teacher. He also vicariously identifies with the teacher's work
problems. Usually, the principal has failed to help his teacher
with problems in areas where he is also in conflict. Since he is
once removed from the direct consultation, he gains relief and
help with his problems without their ever being made explicit.
Subsequently, he may communicate what he has learned to other
teachers and even to fellow administrators. This is especially
true of problems concerned with authority and the acceptance of
one's own limitations—areas of special concern to administrators.

Experienced consultants have come to recognize how often
teacher-consultees present the problems they are unable to deal
with by behaving toward the consultant as their difficult students
have behaved toward them. In my experience, this is especially
true in instances of hostile, provocative behavior, or when the
incessant demands of one or more students for exclusive attention
have exhausted the teacher. The teacher finds himself in conflict
about what is fair to the demanding student, to the class, and lastly,
if at all, to himself. These teachers may come to consultation with
hostile, demanding, provocative attitudes, and sometimes belligerent pounding at the consultant for answers to their problems. One
senses the teacher-consultee's wary, anxious observation of the
consultant and the close scrutiny of his methods as he handles this
situation. In these instances there is the clearest identification
with the consultant and incorporation of his attitudes and methods
of handling problems.

In almost all mental health consultation, identification with the
consultant and incorporation of his attitudes and methods of working with problems are part of the process of ego integration. From
my point of view, mental health consultation is essentially conducted at the ego level. In my own work during the past twelve years,
I have tried to apply the growing insights from ego psychology to
refine the consultation process. These insights include an awareness of the integrative capacities in all human beings, even those
who are very sick; efforts to understand the individual's malintegrative behavior in the current situation and to assess that
behavior in terms of the current realities; a detailed examination
of the problems so that through attention to the minute details of
the current difficulties in functioning one may begin to elucidate
methods of resolution usually inherent in the troubles; help in the
resolution of conflicts by honest assessment of the reality facing
the person and a step-by-step analysis of the ways in which certain obstacles to resolution were noted, understood, and handled
by the person. Thus the consultant is task-oriented; this helps
reduce the regressive helplessness of the consultee and enlists
him as a collaborator, not a patient, to work together with the

consultant to resolve the particular work problems. The consultant's understanding of the consultee's neurotic conflicts, which make for his work problems, is used to find the dynamically appropriate comments which will help reduce the central anxieties and permit the collaboration to occur.

Inherent in all of this is an underlying thesis in ego psychology: that the conflict between unconscious forces results from malintegrative experiences during infancy and childhood. These conflicts usually become manifest as a struggle between regression and helplessness on one side, and mastery and integrative, productive behavior on the other. In consultative situations involving rebellious feelings and behavior toward authority, these aspects are perhaps most clearly seen. The consultee may begin by presenting his own problems of helplessness in handling hostile or rebellious behavior in his students and then go on to talk of his anger and hatred toward the unfair, punitive administrator. In such comments the genesis of the conflicts in early experience often becomes clear. If, after listening carefully, one returns to a close examination of the classroom events with inquiries about how the teacher handles other classroom problems, one gets a sense of the capacity for effective teaching that is present. A detailed assessment of the actual problems with the rebellious student often gives clues to the teacher's momentary awareness of choices at critical points of dealing with the youngster—choices that were not heeded, so that the helpless, regressive feeling overwhelmed the teacher and created the resulting havoc. At this point some effort to externalize the situation by using experiences of the consultant or others may illustrate why such moments of choice are difficult to detect and to use, and how one's anger with authority may make such work more difficult. Finally, one can illustrate that other solutions might be possible if these critical moments were recognized and then handled differently.

The strategies and tactics of mental health consultation, when examined, are based upon application of theoretical constructs from psychoanalytic thinking and practice. Such application of theory to areas of practice outside the dyadic relationship are a constant challenge to the mental health worker.

PREVENTIVE ASPECTS OF
MENTAL HEALTH CONSULTATION TO SCHOOLS*

I. N. Berlin

The vast increase in numbers of emotionally disturbed children, adolescents, and adults is dramatically illustrated by the swelling ranks of nonlearners in schools; unabating delinquency, violence, and pregnancies among adolescents; and increased divorce rates and decreased job and interpersonal satisfactions among adults. All these have made society increasingly conscious of psychological problems and the need for treatment. Studies have indicated that there will never be enough mental health professionals to give treatment to the children who need it, not to mention the disturbed adult population. Prevention must concern us as one attack on this overwhelming problem.

In the schools we are concerned more with secondary than with primary prevention (5). The prenatal, early infancy, and childhood problems antedate school—problems that may stem from the mother's depression, from parental conflicts that affect the infant and small child, from mother-infant and mother-toddler alienation; or from the mother's personality problems or inexperience in the mothering process. Similarly, problems may be caused by the unhappy child's reaction to his environment, to neurophysiological dysfunction, or to sociocultural deprivation which, in a vicious circle, increases the child's turmoil and thereby increases family troubles. All these have already had their effects by the time the child enters kindergarten or first grade. There are, however, a few areas of primary prevention in which educators do play a vital role, especially in cases of crisis in a child's life, in which an educator's sensitivity and response to the child may be of crucial importance.

Secondary prevention centers around the early identification of emotional disturbance due to interpersonal, neurophysiological, or

---

*Reprinted with permission from Mental Hygiene, 51:34, 1967.

sociocultural factors, and early intervention by the educator through the mental health consultation process. In many instances this process includes involving the parents; in a few instances referral must be made to community resources. However, preventive work centers essentially around learning to recognize and to use the potentially healing or therapeutic aspects of the educative process. Prevention also depends on the alertness of educators to normal maturational and school crises that may affect the vulnerable child adversely if they are not recognized, understood, and reacted to helpfully.

Our concern here is with some general aspects of prevention in schools, the role of mental health consultation as a means of facilitating and enhancing prevention, and a specific technique or method of mental health consultation found effective by some mental health specialists and educators.

Most teachers are capable of recognizing early behavioral disturbances due to emotional factors, or a child's inability to learn because of maturational lag, sociocultural deprivation, or manifestations of brain dysfunction. Bowers (4) and others have compared the reliability of teachers' concerns and evaluations of a child's functioning in school with later diagnostic studies by mental health professionals and have found teachers' observations very trustworthy. Thus, the early recognition of a child's problems in school is possible.

The central problems are subsequent assessment of the disturbance by educators and others in terms of the child's sociocultural background, neuromuscular maturation, emotional instability, and possible organic retardation. Once a tentative diagnosis is made, the experienced educator can begin to make some prognoses and attempt to verify them by observations in the classroom. He may then be better able to decide whether a youngster needs further, prompt evaluation. Inherent in the process of early identification of problems is contact with the parents to obtain their observations on the child and his development, and to assess any evident troubles in and between parents that may be affecting the child.

It needs to be stressed and re-stressed that, even when evaluation and treatment are undertaken by outside agencies, the school still has the challenging problem of determining how educative methods and classroom experiences can be used to take maximal advantage of the early recognition of disturbance and to enhance the therapeutic process. Since treatment is a slow process, it requires all the additional help possible in the everyday life of the child. Mental health consultation is often helpful in developing collaboration between the educator and the psychotherapist. The consultant is also able to help educators recognize that learning expectations are often supportive to the sick child's ego.

MATURATIONAL CRISES OF THE SCHOOL-AGE CHILD

Leaving the protection of home and mother at the age of five or six years represents a crisis for some children. How the school deals with the child and parents, and with the child's fear of school and desire to stay home, can affect the prevention of future disability.

Restriction of gross motor activity, which is a prerequisite for attending to the teacher and to seat work, and learning how to learn, may precipitate a crisis, especially for slowly maturing boys who are not yet able to contain large muscle activity in favor of the pleasures to be obtained from increased fine motor coordination. The recognition of these problems and of the crisis that may result from pushing a child and not providing frequent outlets for large muscle movement and suitable rewards for sitting still, using small muscles, and acquiring fine motor coordination, is important to the learning future of the child.

The use of imaginative stimulation of all the senses and of special educational techniques to help the socioculturally deprived child achieve learning readiness is among the educator's most important preventive activities. The third grade—in which learning commences with real seriousness and most children are maturationally ready to learn—may find many children still unable to read, poorly motivated to learn, and unable to sit still, yet wanting to learn and to experience the fun of learning and the excitement of acquiring knowledge so evident in their classmates. The educator's failure to recognize increased hyperactivity, truculence, and opposition to learning as evidence of possible acute conflict between the desire to learn and the inability to find the means of learning may aggravate this crisis and alienate the child from the learning process and its potential satisfactions.

Similarly, it is often difficult for educators to keep in mind the fact that, for most youngsters, any sudden spurt in growth means that energy is being mobilized for the growing process and that there may be less energy available for learning. Thus, the correlation of growth spurts with falling-off in grades points to a need for increased understanding of the youngster rather than pressure for performance, but without permitting a serious drop in performance. Usually, vigorous engagement in learning returns in a few weeks.

In early adolescence, the development of secondary sexual characteristics, growth spurts, and the flowering of social activities—especially for girls—often result in reduced energy for learning.

The shift from elementary school to the middle school or junior high school, in which the child has many teachers instead of one, may present crises for particular children who emotionally need the support, the firm expectations, and the rewards of a single parental figure. These children may begin to do badly in the larger and more impersonal junior high school, and may need to form a tie with a central person to facilitate their adaptation.

If the situation is correctly assessed and dealt with, each of these potential crises offers the educator opportunities to help a youngster mobilize his integrative capabilities and learn to cope more effectively with the external world.

Preventive Implications of Students' Life Crises

Many children, in the course of their school experiences, undergo serious crises in their family situations that may require alert aid from the teacher in order to prevent serious impairment of the child's mental health. For example, death or divorce of parents; death of siblings or other family members; unemployment of the father; instability in the parents' financial or emotional support; serious illness of, or accident to, the student or another member of the family, with its potentially ominous import—all may have a marked impact on the child.

Perhaps the best single indicator of a serious crisis in a child's life is an abrupt change in behavior, such as a sudden loss of interest in learning, withdrawal from social interaction, explosive behavior (i.e., "blowing up" or crying), or silence and isolation on the part of a hyperactive child. Such changes should be a signal for inquiry. In these instances, the continued interest and support of teachers and others may be a vital factor in the child's ability to deal with the home crises. All experienced teachers can site examples of how their support and, sometimes, intervention have been important to a child's emotional survival during a crisis in which the child felt alone and helpless. Here, also, the mental health consultant may be helpful in finding the best ways for a teacher to approach a difficult and non-relating child.

The Therapeutic Effect of Learning

In order to be an effective adult in our technical society, the child must master ever more difficult and complex subject matter and acquire a variety of increasingly more refined skills. Mastery of academic materials depends on the satisfaction, pleasures, and rewards of the learning process. These often have not been acquired in the preschool years if the child has lived with deprived, troubled, not very effective, and not very nurturant or supportive parents. The school's efforts to help a child learn, through a variety of sensory experiences and pleasurable early learning experiences, may begin to help him to develop habits and successes in learning that can be critical to his future living as an effective adult. Thus, inherent in the learning process itself are preventive and therapeutic implications, which the mental health consultant may be able to help the teacher make more explicit for particular children.

THE ROLE OF THE MENTAL HEALTH CONSULTANT IN SCHOOLS

The mental health consultant in a school is usually a social worker, clinical psychologist, or psychiatrist employed by the administration. This consultant may be helpful in the school in a variety of ways, depending upon the needs of the school, its personnel, and the skill and experience of the consultant himself (1,2).

First, he may be of factual help. He may provide information about growth and development, the impact of certain sociocultural experiences, diagnostic implications of a particular type of behavior of child or parents, or the community resources available for diagnosis or treatment of particular children.

Second, he may be of interpretive help. His knowledge of interpersonal dynamics and the developmental process may permit him to piece together the data gathered by the teacher, the administrator, the school nurse, and others, and to give some picutre of the origins of, and reasons for, the child's difficulties. He may be able to draw implications from the child's present behavior and past experiences for corrective classroom experiences. He may be able to delineate what the child may need from an adult that the teacher can give as part of his job as educator.

Third, the consultant may be of help in clarifying the integrative part that learning may play in the child's life and in the reduction of the child's troubles. He may be able to help teachers recognize that emotional disturbance, and even severe mental illness, may be benefited by the teacher's firm expectation that a child can learn and, through learning, feel more effective and intact. He may a'
be able to trace the non-integrative experiences of the distr
hostile, hyperactive child, so that the teacher can begin t
nize the kind of attitudes—the personal investment, st
concerned firmness, persistence, and rewards—re
particular child begin to learn. He may also b
educator become alert and sensitized to certa

behavior that indicate—often through negative and challenging behavior—the child's increased readiness for certain expectations, for increased tolerance of closeness, or for more firmness, as required by the child to take the next step in learning and personality integration.

Fourth, the consultant may be in a position to help the educator preserve his own mental health in the face of the many pressing mental health problems of his students and the students' parents. He may be able to aid the educator with his own self-expectations, which are often inconsistent with the harsh realities. Thus, he may assist the teacher who feels he is a failure if his youngsters are not up to grade or if he is unable to generate in his students responsive pleasure and excitement in learning. By enabling the teacher to recognize the obstacles to learning and the therapeutic function of learning for certain children, the consultant may encourage him to find satisfaction in the bite-size increments of learning that occur as children begin to work through the initial turmoil of the learning process. He may help the teacher recognize, with more and more genuine pleasure and satisfaction, the learning and consequent changes that occur as the teacher provides the appropriate milieu for change. He may also be in a position to interpret the pressures of the community and administration for heroic action, so that the teacher sees the realities of his day-to-day job in terms of an accumulation of tiny increments of learning and behavior change.

Hopefully, the consultant can also aid the teacher, under the trying conditions of very difficult classrooms, to recognize his human feelings of despair, anger, and even hate, as well as a sort of general guilt at not being able to love all the children and work miracles for them. When she or he understands these as common human feelings, the teacher often feels less frustrated and is able to work more effectively bit by bit and day by day. A not-so-incidental result of this is that the teacher provides an example to his students of what they need to do, showing that achievement comes not with wishing, but with hard and unremitting work. As the teacher evaluates the reality of his situation more objectively and scales down his self-expectations, he begins to try to clarify where each student is and what he needs to learn. He then begins to expect realistic increments of learning from each student. And, as his students do learn more under these conditions, he feels better about himself and his job.

Inherent in all this is a serious problem. Mental health consultation is designed to help educators deal more effectively with disturbed children in the schools rather than get rid of them. The reality of the situation is this: there is nowhere to refer all the roblems and no way to wash one's hands of them, since there are so many problem children. Educators must understand the function of consultation—to help teachers learn to work with more children more effectively so that only the most seriously disturbed youngsters will require referral.

A METHOD OF MENTAL HEALTH CONSULTATION

There are four or five steps in the process of mental health consultation—often not consecutive steps, but all important to successful consultation (3). Perhaps the most important guideline is that the process is designed to promote collaboration between educator and mental health specialist, with the goal of helping the former to do a better job with students who have mental health problems.

The first step is the consultant's effort to become acquainted with the organization, structure, and problems of schools in general; the usual burdens of the teacher; and the special problems of the particular school. The consultant must become sufficiently immersed in the school setting so that he can understand the teacher's comments in the context of the special milieu in which the teacher works.

The second step centers around the consultant's efforts to facilitate the educator's acceptance of the mental health consultant as a potentially helpful person, rather than one who is concerned with analyzing the educator and uncovering character problems and unconscious motivations. In short, the consultant's concern is the educator's work problems, and not his personal ones. The educator should experience the mental health consultant as a fellow human being whose task is to engage him as a collaborator, not in any way as a patient or client.

This phase of the work may take some time. The working-through is focused on the consultant's trying to indicate, in a variety of ways, that he can understand the teacher's feelings about the particular students he teaches in his particular setting. The consultant's projection of empathy with, and acceptance of, the teacher's feelings as both human and understandable should lead to collaboration in the service of the student.

The third stage of consultation is concerned with relieving the anxieties, self-recriminations, and feelings of failure that result from attempting to teach difficult and disturbed children. The reduction of teacher anxiety is a prerequisite to being able to explore methods of working with the child. Unless the educator's self-blame, tension, and feeling that he should be able to handle such problems without help are dealt with, he is not able to listen to, and consider, alternative courses of action. Teacher anxiety is best reduced by

the consultant's discussing similar problems that he or others have
been confronted with, thus clearly demonstrating his understanding
of similar feelings and moments of impasse.

For example, the teacher who has to deal with hostile, aggressive, hyperactive children knows that I understand her problems
when I describe some harrowing experiences of my own in a playroom with a child who had similar problems; but I have had to contend with only one youngster for one hour once or twice a week,
rather than with 36 children daily for six or seven hours. Since I,
too, have experienced the kind of wounds that come from being
rendered temporarily ineffectual by a child, teachers seem to know
from my comments that I understand their feelings.

The fourth step is an effort to increase the teacher's distance
from the problem and his objectivity by using all the data provided
to draw a picture of the etiology of a particular child's problems,
showing how experience with the important adults in the child's
life has affected him and resulted in his present behavior. This
not only helps the teacher feel less responsible for the child's
problems and for his immediate cure, but also indicates the conditions in which the child's problems developed and where it may
be necessary to take hold, or what adult behavior is required to
alter the child's view of the adult and of himself. In instances of
sociocultural deprivation, it may also help the teacher to understand that, as a teacher, he has an important function in the community. Not only does he help children become more effective
persons, but also, by participating in community activities, he may
enhance his access to parents in the service of their children.

The fifth step is considering alternative methods of dealing with
the child's behavior that, in the consultant's own experience or that
of other educators, have been effective. Often the consultant's understanding of the origin of the child's problems can be restated to the
educator so that, from this, certain attitudes, attentions, and expectations seem to evolve for mutual consideration. Alternative
possibilities congruent with the the teacher's experience and ideas
need to be explored. The consultant who makes a recommendation
or gives a prescription instead of fostering a consideration of
alternatives usually learns that the teacher has already tried what
he proposes and found that it did not work; or, if the teacher tacitly
accepts a recommendation to which he has not contributed, he is
apt to report back the next time that it has not been effective. Thus,
the consultant needs not only to help the educator consider alternatives, but also to suggest that these be tentatively tried and reported on the next time for mutual reconsideration.

The sixth step is the follow-up of consultation, in which sustained interest, concern, and supportive help provide a recurrent oppor-

tunity for the teacher to learn to deal with his problems more effectively.

Inherent in all of these phases of consultation is the probability that much of the effect of the process results from the identification of the educator with the consultant, his attitudes, and his methods of interaction. The consultant's attitudes, which are based on respect for the teacher as a potentially effective collaborator who can learn to use teaching and learning as a means of helping disturbed students, are often adopted by the teacher. Very clearly, teachers often act toward their difficult students as consultants have acted toward them.

In my own work, I have felt it important that the administrator be present. As the key person in the school, he not only needs to agree that the ideas to be tried are consonant with his own philosophy, but also to mediate between teacher and consultant. In addition, the administrator can learn from observing the consultation process what aspects of it he can use to make his own work more effective.

Each successful consultation not only reduces the child's present learning and behavior disturbance, but also prevents future learning disability and personality disorder. The youngster's increased learning ability and effectiveness in school may change his view of himself and his functioning in the world. The teacher is frequently able to apply what he has learned in consultation about one child to other children in the classroom. The consultation process thus helps the teacher to feel ever more effective and successful as a teacher, and furthers the goal of prevention through both pupil and teacher.

REFERENCES

1. BERLIN, I. N. Ment. Hygiene, 40:215, 1956.
2. BERLIN, I. N. J. Amer. Acad. Child Psychiat., 1:671, 1962.
3. BERLIN, I. N. Ment. Hygiene, 43:257, 1964.
4. BOWERS, E. M. Early identification of emotionally handicapped children in school. Springfield, Ill.: Charles C Thomas, 1960.
5. EISENBERG, L., & GRUENBERG, E. M. Amer. J. Orthopsychiat., 31:355, 1961.

INDEX*

*Underscored page number indicates bibliographic reference.

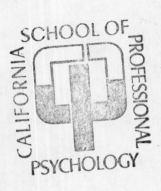

CALIFORNIA SCHOOL OF PROFESSIONAL PSYCHOLOGY